'Very easy to read and informative.'
– Dr Yehudi Gordon, author and renowned gynaeocologist

'Claudia Spahr has written a wise, informative and entertaining
pregnancy and birth guide that is perfect for both older mothers
and equally relevant if you're still in your teens or twenties. Don't miss
this one!'
– Ina May Gaskin, author and founder of The Farm Midwifery Centre

'At last a book that puts the risk factors into perspective and
encourages older women to become mothers! Claudia Spahr offers a
treasure trove of useful guidance about the wonderful options there are
for a positive and life-changing pregnancy at any age. Written with a
twist of humour, this book will inspire and inform as much as it will
amuse you.'
– Janet Balaskas, Founder Active Birth and pregnancy yoga pioneer

'I'm glad there's finally a book I can hand to all the terrified women
who come to me in their thirties. *Right Time Baby* is just the right
medicine for women who want to have a baby but who have been led
to believe that their fertile time is drawing to a close. Nothing could
be further from the truth. Take heart, read this book and tap into your
fertility birthright.'
– Christiane Northrup, MD, author of *Women's Bodies, Women's Wisdom*
and *The Wisdom of Menopause*

'The book by Claudia Spahr is perfectly adapted to our time because
many sentences end with a question mark. Delayed motherhood is
an unprecedented situation on the five continents. When facing new
situations the priority is to phrase new questions.'
– Dr Michel Odent, author and founder of the
Primal Health Research Centre

'A book like this is needed because more women are waiting to have
children. The concerns for them are different, so by being more focused
this book will be particularly relevant for them.'
– Marilyn Glenville, author and renowned fertility expert

D1041394

'This book gives women a timely and positive understanding
that pregnancy over 35 is not just a possibility, but a source of joy
and delight. Claudia offers oodles of useful tips and helpful information,
presented in a really accessible and down-to-earth manner.
A fabulously helpful resource.'
– Uma Dinsmore-Tuli, author and pregnancy yoga pioneer

'The time is right for a book like this. I shall be recommending
*Right Time Baby* to all my pregnant clients.'
– Dr Jonathon Dao, ND OMD

# Right Time Baby

Claudia Spahr

HAY HOUSE

Australia • Canada • Hong Kong • India
South Africa • United Kingdom • United States

First published and distributed in the United Kingdom by:
Hay House UK Ltd, 292B Kensal Rd, London W10 5BE. Tel.: (44) 20 8962 1230;
Fax: (44) 20 8962 1239. www.hayhouse.co.uk

Published and distributed in the United States of America by:
Hay House, Inc., PO Box 5100, Carlsbad, CA 92018-5100. Tel.: (1) 760 431 7695 or
(800) 654 5126; Fax: (1) 760 431 6948 or (800) 650 5115. www.hayhouse.com

Published and distributed in Australia by:
Hay House Australia Ltd, 18/36 Ralph St, Alexandria NSW 2015. Tel.: (61) 2 9669 4299;
Fax: (61) 2 9669 4144. www.hayhouse.com.au

Published and distributed in the Republic of South Africa by:
Hay House SA (Pty), Ltd, PO Box 990, Witkoppen 2068. Tel./Fax: (27) 11 467 8904.
www.hayhouse.co.za

Published and distributed in India by:
Hay House Publishers India, Muskaan Complex, Plot No.3, B-2, Vasant Kunj, New Delhi
– 110 070. Tel.: (91) 11 4176 1620; Fax: (91) 11 4176 1630. www.hayhouse.co.in

Distributed in Canada by:
Raincoast, 9050 Shaughnessy St, Vancouver, BC V6P 6E5. Tel.: (1) 604 323 7100;
Fax: (1) 604 323 2600

© Claudia Spahr, 2011

The moral rights of the author have been asserted.

The author of this book does not dispense medical advice or prescribe the use of any
technique as a form of treatment for physical or medical problems without the advice
of a physician, either directly or indirectly. The intent of the author is only to offer
information of a general nature to help you in your quest for emotional and spiritual
wellbeing. In the event you use any of the information in this book for yourself, which is
your constitutional right, the author and the publisher assume no responsibility for your
actions.

A catalogue record for this book is available from the British Library.

ISBN 978-1-84850-256-7

Printed and bound in the UK by
CPI Mackays, Chatham ME5 8TD

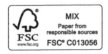

*For Javier, mi amor, who made me a mother.*
*For Santiago*
*and all other Right Time Babies.*
*May your futures be filled with wisdom and love.*

# Contents

# *Acknowledgements*

My sincerest thanks to all the wonderful women, mothers and parents who shared their intimate and personal stories for this book. I would also like to thank all the doctors and experts for their time and key insights, without which this guide would not be as relevant. Thanks also to the team at Hay House who – like a good mother – provided me with a nurturing base and gave me the freedom to fly.

# *Preface*

A book of this scope requires a substantial amount of research and investigation. Apart from reading material on everything from fertility to child-rearing, I conducted countless interviews. These included world authorities and experts on fertility, pregnancy, childbirth and women's health: people such as Michel Odent, Ina May Gaskin and Christiane Northrup. Where possible I met the experts in person, otherwise the interviews were conducted by telephone. I also did face-to-face interviews with 50 mothers, who all had their children after the age of 35. These interviews gave me insight into the range of concerns and issues that affect later mothers. I have used quotes from these experts and mothers throughout the book.

I also collected information and statistics via a qualitative study: a survey I sent out with 30 questions. Sixty women filled in the questionnaire and added their comments. I decided against posting the survey in an anonymous chat-room, in order to keep it manageable and less susceptible to error. I do believe the answers are representative for this age group, and that having a larger number of participants would have provided a similar outcome.

As for the book, you'll see that I sometimes refer to the baby as 'he' and sometimes 'she' to avoid being gender specific or using cumbersome 'he or she' formulations. I have also referred to the baby in the singular even though you may have twins. I often talk about a 'partner' or 'husband' although I'm well aware that many women are single or don't have a male partner, so please don't feel excluded by this assumption. This book is also for you.

Although the advice I give is generally backed up by more than one source – a habit I picked up as a news journalist – it will not replace any medical treatment you might need. If in doubt, do consult a good doctor. I have added links for further reading in the Bibliography and References. However, not all studies or resources are listed, simply because this would have taken up far too many pages of an already long book. If you have questions about anything I mention, feel free to contact me via my website.

# *Introduction*

Is there ever a right time to have a baby?

In our twenties we're discovering ourselves and the world. Many of us pursue some form of higher education and are busy turning jobs into careers. We want to have fun, be free, party all night and sleep all day. There's nothing as exhilarating as being young and independent with life laid out before you like a red carpet. Having a baby would get in the way, it would tie you down and to someone – at least that's what I thought. No one was going to steal my youth from me. And there was still so much to learn, and so much insecurity.

Then you turn 30. You've had a few proper relationships, your heart's been broken and you've learned that nothing lasts forever. But you're also more at ease, smarter, sexier and likely to be having the time of your life. Sometimes you feel a little disorientated and looking for some deeper meaning or purpose. Often this is found in work; the early thirties are those intense years where you dedicate everything to *getting somewhere*. There may be a man around, but he expresses even less interest in committing to family than you do.

Suddenly you're in your mid-thirties and it's time to procreate. Not because you've achieved everything you want in life, or visited all the places you want to see – but simply because everyone says you should get a move on. That perfect window of opportunity for a baby has been and gone and your body is already on the downward spiral – allegedly. Time is ticking. You and your ovaries are getting old. Panic sets in. You might have a partner or husband, but they're still not ready. So what do you do? Dump them and find someone else? You might be single and looking, but the best catches are either taken or running from you. Did anyone think of telling them to hurry up and find a nice woman to shack up and breed with? What about your job? Would there even be space in your life for motherhood *and* making money?

These are the paradoxes for females of childbearing age in our modern society; so much to do but never enough time to do it all.

And what about those dream babies? What kind of mothers do they need?

Delaying childbearing in order to achieve a better balance in life – be it to find yourself or the right partner, or to build your career – can only be beneficial for a child. Life experience transfers well to mothering skills; you have more stability, confidence and patience. Increased life expectancy means you should be around long enough to watch your children grow old themselves. Most of us are vibrant and energetic well into our forties. Definitely not too old to do what we always thought we would one day: get pregnant and have a healthy baby.

Or, you may already have children – maybe from an earlier relationship – and worry that it will be different this time because you're older.

There's plenty you can do to improve health, with enough scientific evidence now linking the right nutrition with good health. Taking an informed, active role in your own healthcare is probably the key to becoming a later parent. But health is far more than just physical; it includes our thoughts, emotions and spiritual path. If we're in balance we have the remarkable capacity to fight disease and self-heal. Louise L. Hay, bestselling author and founder of Hay House, the publishers of this guide, says 'The thoughts you choose to think and the foods you choose to eat are everything to do with your health.'

As a journalist I was taught to *look behind the mirror*, and as a writer it's my role to question the status quo. There are plenty of books on the market which give you the standard advice on pregnancy and motherhood; but there is so much more. That is where this book is different. I have included the latest research from exciting new subjects like cell biology, foetal origins, quantum physics and neuroscience. I've also incorporated the most contemporary ideas from psychology and nutrition. This means there's a lot of 'what the doctor doesn't tell you' in this book, so you can get the whole picture and be in charge. Once you're a mother you'll probably just want the best for your child. The best isn't always what the pharmaceutical lobby recommends or popular culture sees fit. When a baby is born, it has very simple needs, which every mother is able to fulfil. It's worth remembering there are societies where there are no birth inductions, no cot deaths, no postnatal depression and no temper tantrums for the 'terrible twos'.

I wrote this book with one main goal: to empower women to embrace motherhood positively, regardless of their age. In this guide you should find appreciation and understanding for the massive transformation you're going through. I also wrote it to stimulate and encourage you to make new choices. The advice is what an informed girlfriend would share with you – the nerdy one who likes reading heavy science books and then summarizes the message for you in 2 minutes. That's why I spent months interviewing experts and other mothers, trawling through books, libraries, articles and medical journals in order to condense important information for your convenience. I wrote the book I would have wanted to read before I became a mother, and I can assure you I will be putting these insights into practice for further 'baby making' at the ripe old age of 42.

This book was also written to entertain you. Motherhood is serious business and a sense of humour is more vital than ever.

Do remember: every woman, every child and every situation is different. After you've read *Right Time Baby* and gathered any extra information you feel is important, it would be my greatest wish that you recognize and honour your own instincts and the innate wisdom of your baby. Then this book will have fulfilled its purpose and you'll have the best guide you'll ever need.

# CHAPTER 1

# *Are You Ready?*

## ALL CHANGE

Motherhood is a journey into the unknown. It's an irreversible transformation I've never heard anyone regret. With the birth of every baby, a mother is also born; and a mother she'll remain, for the rest of her life. Venturing on this journey later in your life – when you know more about who you are – is an exciting time for it to happen. The change is likely to be more radical than for a younger woman who matures with her children.

No matter how you approach motherhood, a child alters your priorities. In fact, it completely takes over your life – especially in the intense first year. You can wave goodbye to self-indulgence (and anything else beginning with *self*) because your metamorphosis from 'me' to 'mum' puts you firmly at the bottom of the pecking order, and your little mite way up there at the top, before anybody else – including your rather neglected partner. Having a child heralds the beginning of a lifelong relationship with a human being tied to you by blood; the strongest bond of all.

Weird stuff happens when we become parents. We worry more and we cry more, especially when we see vulnerable little children or animals in need of care. Many of us turn into our own parents – at least for a while – and start fussing unnecessarily. I transformed into a worrier AND a wimp. Previously fearless to the point of bungee jumping from a cable-car suspended above a waterfall, I now get anxious just sitting in the passenger seat when my partner drives (admittedly he's a Latin who gets occasional attacks of road rage). Becoming a mother does very good things to you, too. It makes you effortlessly happy and fulfilled. You discover a new kind of love – one that never runs out or expects anything in return.

Motherhood is one of the most instinctive desires we have and the socio-cultural pressure is overwhelming – if all your friends are procreating, it can make you feel quite left out being childless. Being a mum is not something we absolutely need to experience to understand what it means to be female, of course, but the miracle of pregnancy and birth and the absolute joy of holding a newborn baby in your arms makes everything else pale in comparison. Apart from fulfilling our basic purpose to perpetuate life, it's what makes the world go round.

## WHY THE DELAY?

*Mama Said*

The skills we've acquired to make choices in daily life don't apply to breeding. As the first generation of women with the 'shall I, shan't I have a baby?' dilemma, we had little in the way of role models to nudge us in the right direction. Most of our mothers didn't get to choose. They fought hard for liberation but were unable to fully benefit themselves. Held back by glass ceilings, domestic duties and school runs, they spent free evenings at Tupperware parties rather than networking dos. Instead of realizing their own potential, they projected their hopes and dreams onto us – the bright young daughters. We studied, we travelled, we enjoyed and we worked; harder and often better than the men. The subliminal hum in the corridors of corporate land confirmed what our mothers had experienced: careers and carrycots do not go together well. So we waited until the time was better. But the perfect time to have a baby never arrives.

Not only our mothers, but anyone with an opinion would suggest putting off having children at the most fertile age. We were told to get a career (more than *just* a job) and not settle for the first best man who came along. The young women in today's tough, consumer world are less idealistic, so maybe we really are the last generation to harbour romantic fantasies.

## Waiting for Mr Right

Most of us are independent and fussy; so fussy we spend our 'best years' looking for the perfect partner with whom to have our dream baby. The *trying out potential fathers* process is fun for a while, but eventually it becomes tiring, frustrating and heartbreaking. The men we temporarily shack up with are grown-up youths like us, eons away from developing their nesting instincts. And if you do reach the 'I want to have your baby' stage with one because your clock is ticking louder than his – then the mere glint of that desire in your eyes is enough to send him packing. The majority of males we take to our beds are just not good enough as father material. And why should we accept second best? We were told *it has to be perfect*. So we look for an upgrade. We surf for a soulmate. The next best thing could be just around the corner. And often shows up a decade late.

For most of us a sense of urgency kicks in around 35 – the age when Carrie in *Sex and the City* claims she is 'officially old'. A friend of mine finished with her long-term partner after being told by her gynaecologist that she should be thinking about getting pregnant. Armed with this information she cornered her mate, who expressed no desire to breed this side of 40. Her reason for breaking up is a classic for women in their mid-thirties. But the countdown often starts even earlier. There's a scene in *Friends* where Rachel dumps her boyfriend at her 30th birthday party. She announces she wants to have children by 35, and calculates that she should already be with the guy she's going to marry, if she wants this five-year plan to work.

> An interesting but not particularly surprising result from my *Right Time Baby* survey showed that the majority of women delayed childbearing because of taking time to find the right man.

Madonna was a rebellious role model for many women of my generation. She got pregnant with her first child, Lourdes, aged 38. A comfortable ten years younger, I pinned the newspaper clipping announcing her pregnancy to my noticeboard to remind myself that I still had a good decade to live to the full; another ten years until it was 'time'. Life was good – far too good to want to change anything. Today, I can happily say my oracle came true. At 39 I got pregnant and had my first child 2 months before hitting 40. You could suggest I 'programmed' my cells – and they delivered!

## Gap Mothers

As women get healthier and live longer, they're more confident about becoming mothers later. A further modern phenomenon is the 'gap mother', who has a child at least ten years after her last one. With nearly 50 per cent of all marriages ending in divorce, many people remarry or form 'second' relationships. Half of all couples in second relationships or remarriages go on to have a child.

Having a nestling grow out of nappies, getting him through maths exams and acne and then starting all over again with another one (while the big one displays pubescent behaviour) can be challenging. However, a baby can really bond a family together; older children develop their own special relationship with a new sibling. And remember: babysitters don't come cheap these days. A toddler needing attention is a great way to keep a teenager occupied and off the DX. You can actually go to the toilet by yourself because trustworthy arms are there to hold pint-size.

## Some Mature Mum Pros

Having children later comes with lots of advantages; especially for the kids:

1. **Healthier babies**
   A study at the University of Texas showed that older mothers had healthier babies than younger mothers.[1]

2. **Proactive healthcare seekers**
   86 per cent of a study group of pregnant women over 35 were found to promote health through nutritional intake, lifestyle and rest patterns. They conscientiously eliminated harmful substances and altered exercise, employment and daily responsibilities to accommodate pregnancy.[2]

3. **Better moods**
   An Italian study showed that women over 35 displayed less somatic tension, less anxiety and a greater feeling of exuberance and vigour during pregnancy.[3]

4. **Later mothers breastfeed more**
   Due to informed decisions and more available time, the later mother is proven to breastfeed her child for longer.[4]

5.  **Fewer baby blues**
    Studies show that mature mums are less prone to postnatal depression than women who have their children at a younger age.[5]

6.  **More time for the children**
    Research confirms that older parents have more available time to spend with their children.[6]

7.  **More money for the children**
    Studies show older parents have fewer children and improved resources to be shared by them.[7]

8.  **Children have higher IQs**
    A study based on 4,300 older mothers found their children to perform better at school and be better behaved.[8] The authors of the study said the reasons could be biological – older mothers made sure they had better nutrition during pregnancy – and social: their home environment was more conducive to learning.

9.  **Older mothers live longer**
    Numerous studies[9] show that having children later in life increases the lifespan of the mother; in fact a woman who gives birth over the age of 40 is four times more likely to reach the age of 100. The prime age for childbearing, in terms of maternal health and longevity, allegedly lies between 34 and 40.

## Some Personal Lifestyle Advantages

A later mum is generally more settled and ready in herself to have a baby. She has increased maturity to deal with all the emotional and financial aspects, and thus creates a more stable environment for the baby to grow up in. Many later mothers agree they are better parents than they would have been in younger years – with more wisdom, time and patience to devote to their child.[10]

According to my survey, women found the advantages of later motherhood outweighed the disadvantages. They felt more ready to focus on family because they hadn't missed out on independence and didn't mind giving up some freedom. Some 63 per cent said it was the perfect time for a baby, and 9 per cent said they would have waited even longer.

## Some Expert Opinions

*'Many women who have a baby later really thrive and make excellent mothers. There are lots of positives; they have good commitment and enjoy their kids; they're financially stable and have a good network of support; they feel better about giving up smoking and late nights to focus on wellbeing and family; they've had a chance to explore other areas of their lives and know they're definitely ready.'*

DR YEHUDI GORDON

*'Many women have their lives more sorted when they're a bit older so they are mentally more prepared for motherhood.'*

ZITA WEST

*'Being older has advantages because you have life experience, maturity, education and a career. Older women are more committed to optimizing health and preparing themselves. They make pregnancy a priority, so it's likely to be a fulfilling experience.'*

JANET BALASKAS

## *And Some Superficial Reasons*

Pregnancy can have a very rejuvenating effect, which is something most of us would welcome. The hormones produced by your body cause your hair to grow faster and thicker, and your nails to become stronger. Due to the increased volume of blood, your cheeks take on an attractive blush – the famous pregnancy *glow* – and your wrinkles soften. Also your breasts *swell,* giving you a more voluptuous vixen look.

> **'When a woman is 20, a child deforms her; when she is 30, he preserves her; and when 40, he makes her young again.'**
>
> LEON BLUM, FRENCH EX-PRIME MINISTER

## AND A FEW DISADVANTAGES

### *Docs' Concerns*

The main disadvantages for older mothers are frequently claimed to be of a medical nature, although considering later mothers are – according to research[11] – 'less likely to engage in risky behaviour' (*now* you tell me!), then these medical risks can be considerably reduced. Go into any bar and see who's on the Chardonnay drip – it's more likely to be the younger woman. In my twenties I would regularly challenge the men in knocking back tequila slammers. This liquid diet continued in my early thirties, when trying out chocolate martinis and cosmopolitans with girlfriends in fancy hotel bars became my favourite indulgence. As for now, well, call me boring, but I get rather thrilled about grinding flaxseeds into fruit smoothies.

> 'It's the best 40th birthday present ever. It's the ideal time to be a mum without a sense of sacrifice that I would have had as a younger mum. My mother said "But why would you want to

breastfeed for so long, you can't go out and have a glass of wine?"
But then, why should I even want to drink? I've spent 20 years
doing that. You wouldn't want to have the lifestyle of a
27-year-old forever."

**CLARE, BABIES AT 40 AND 41**

We live in a culture that's obsessed with talking about risks. Later mothers are constantly warned they've an increased likelihood of having a baby with a birth defect, because this is one risk that allegedly goes up with age. Based on computer statistics, a 40-year-old woman has a 1-in-100 chance of giving birth to a baby with Down's syndrome – but that means she still has a 99 per cent chance of conceiving a healthy baby. Other pregnancy complications sometimes associated with later motherhood, such as diabetes, pre-eclampsia and high blood pressure, are not statistically proven. My own survey showed 83 per cent of mothers had no complications whatsoever, 3 per cent of women had pregnancy diabetes, 2 per cent had pre-eclampsia and 5 per cent had a pre-term baby – figures which are normal for women of *any* age. A US study[12] even showed that women giving birth over 50 didn't have higher health risks than younger women. Nor were they shown to have reduced parenting capacity due to physical or mental ability or parenting stress.

> *'If you exclude the well-known risks there is no spectacular difference in women who have children later; they have just as good a chance of having a healthy baby.'*
>
> DR MICHEL ODENT

Anxiety and negativity are not conducive to a healthy pregnancy, especially now that we know how important the pre-natal period is. Chapter 6 covers all the tests and preoccupations, so that the pregnancy chapters can focus on the more fun bits.

'The main disadvantage I've noticed in being pregnant older is the way others treat you as high risk. There are of course some risk factors, however most older women do very well and the biggest obstacle for them is the expectation of problems just because of their age, and the uncertainty and fear this creates.'

JANET BALASKAS

Another disadvantage often mentioned in connection with later motherhood is a higher chance of miscarriage. Miscarriage affects all women, regardless of age, and the latest research suggests we can do plenty to minimize the risks. All this information is collected in Chapters 2 and 4.

Then there is the whole fertility debate, which is highly fascinating. Infertility is now a worldwide problem affecting everyone, not just the over-35s, partly due to the toxins in our food and environment. The next section, *Misconceptions,* as well as Chapters 2 and 3, talk about ageing and the dreaded decline in fertility.

## Lifestyle Cons

According to my survey, a large number of participants said the main disadvantage of later motherhood was being more tired. However, this is hard to compare. Pregnancy and motherhood tend to be exhausting no matter what age you are. Personally, I tolerate waking up in the middle of the night much better now than as an adolescent-going-on-30 who regularly needed to sleep until lunchtime.

I'd say the main disadvantage of starting procreation later is not being able to have a larger family. You might have an only child or two children spaced quite close together due to the pressure of 'time running out'. It's important to recover well after each pregnancy and birth, which is something mentioned in more detail later in the book.

What surprises a lot of people is that low social class ranks as a higher risk factor in pregnancy than advanced maternal age.

## MISCONCEPTIONS

*Mind Over Matter*

If you're a normal woman growing up in modern society, you're continuously warned about your fertility declining with age. We had a guest at our yoga resort who told me her gynaecologist had suggested she get pregnant soon – she was in her late twenties. Her comment; 'But I'm not ready yet, things are just going well at work and, anyway, I don't even have a boyfriend!' Millions of women in their twenties and thirties are being scared. If you keep hearing that your eggs are getting bad, you start believing it. There's so much talk about the limits we face, rather than the possibilities we could have.

> *'If you see your body as a time bomb, it begins to work on your physiology. These messages are so misguided and damaging to women. From a scientific point of view they increase stress hormones and the way fertility hormones are processed. Your pituitary gland will send signals to the ovaries. We are just beginning to understand the profound effects of belief on our system.'*
> DR CHRISTIANE NORTHRUP

Western science is confirming the premise that your mind controls your health and ageing process. The Harvard professor Ellen Langer successfully proves in her numerous studies that those who free themselves from constricting mindsets can – with only subtle shifts in thinking, language and expectations – look younger and increase longevity.[13] The writer Deepak Chopra also talks about how our thoughts control every cell in the body, and that we have the individual power to influence and postpone ageing.

So if mainstream science has acknowledged that health is largely controlled by our thoughts, wouldn't it make sense that fertility is, too?

In my survey, 68 per cent of later mothers said they felt younger than their age (none said they felt older) – so we can assume these women are all sending positive messages to their bodies. The most surprising result from the questionnaire was just how fast women over 35 – and even over 42 – got pregnant. It took 65 per cent of couples 3 months or less to conceive; much faster than the 8 months it takes on average. Only 15 per cent of couples took longer than 8 months to get pregnant.

There is no clear data proving that it's harder to get pregnant when you're older, even though most doctors will relay it as fact. Like most things, fertility is individual and depends on many variables. To have solid evidence we would have to standardize data, which means comparing like with like. It's difficult to know the true figures of late pregnancy because most women aren't actively trying to conceive in their late forties.

A consequence of the overplayed message about declining fertility is the high abortion rate of the over-40s and even over-50s. In the UK the number of women seeking abortion between the ages of 40 and 44 is identical to that for the under-16s. The Family Planning Association says its evidence suggests most of these were women who just assumed they couldn't get pregnant any more.

## Adapting to Change

When Sheila Kitzinger first published her later motherhood book in 1982 it was called *Birth over Thirty*. Guess what the revised edition, printed in 1994, was called? *Birth over Thirty-Five*. This beautifully displays the shift that's occurred in our society. There have never been so many women having babies in their late thirties and their forties. The average life expectancy of a working-class woman in 1900 was 46 – the age many women today are still vibrant and sexy (debunking yet another stereotype of ten years ago) AND having children. If we are around long enough to see our kids grow up, wouldn't it make sense to be fertile for longer? Cellular division affects the natural ageing process. Old cells cease to replicate, which is why human tissue has a finite lifespan. However, based on normal cellular division, humans should live around 120 years. That's certainly old enough to become a grandmother, even a great-grandmother, if you have your children at 45.

The whole basis of evolution is that, as a species, human beings are highly adaptable. Some scientists argue that menopause is an evolutionary accident of modern life. We used to be dead by the time we hit menopause. It doesn't make biological sense to be reproductive for only a fraction of our lives. Scientists suggest that because the female reproductive system is much more complex than the male's it hasn't caught up or adapted to modern life expectancy yet.[14]

Based on a Sheffield University study, one could speculate that the current trend to have children later means we will evolve into having children at an older age, as longer-lasting fertility genes get passed on.[15]

Here's another interesting fact: the Huichol Indians, descendents of the Aztecs, many of whom live in the remote mountains of North Central Mexico, traditionally have babies well into their forties and fifties. They also enjoy increased longevity. One explanation is that they have different social conditioning to us; another could be their more natural diet and the use of peyote as a medicinal plant.

So here's my prediction: in ten years' time women will be fertile for longer. But this means we must stop brainwashing young women *today* in order for them to 'reprogramme their cells'. And we can de-condition ourselves with more positive messages, starting today.

## HOW WILL A BABY AFFECT MY CAREER?

### *Baby Sabbatical*

One-third of women taking paid maternity leave don't return to work, the main reason being they're unable to work unsuitable hours. Conditions for working parents have improved lately, with more part-time positions, flexi-hours and childcare facilities. However – and this really is a fact of modern life – there's still plenty of discrimination against mothers. It's no surprise that countries like Sweden and Norway – where there are decent maternity and paternity packages – have the highest birth rates in Europe.

> A 30-year study in 18 industrialized countries showed that extending paid maternity leave for new mothers significantly reduced infant mortality. Every 10 weeks of extra maternity leave cuts the infant mortality rate by 2.6 per cent. The infant death rate could be cut by 6.8 per cent in the UK if maternity leave were extended to a year.[16]

Whether you can afford to take time out to care for a baby could be one of the main concerns in the 'shall we breed?' debate. Infants don't necessarily need their mothers ALL the time, but psychologists argue that having two or three consistent carers is better for development. If you feel happier going back to work then there's no reason not to. Feelings of guilt are bound to arise, but as long as you're confident your cherub's being well looked after, there shouldn't be any other hurdles making life harder. And remember, no decisions have to last forever.

A big advantage mature mothers can have is the clout at work to be able to negotiate time off. Many decide to take a baby break because it's the perfect opportunity for family time; or they shift their focus from being primarily career-orientated to being more family-orientated.

'Sometimes people might think I am stuck at home with a baby, but taking a career break was very much a positive decision. I feel that if you are going to wait until 38 to have your first baby, it's not unreasonable to take some time off work to look after it. And quite frankly, after 15 years of working hard, I feel I deserve it. I'm pretty sure that I would not have been able or ready to step back from my career had I had a baby in my twenties.'

KATE, BABIES AT 38 AND 40

## *Homemaking Bliss*

Downsizing to one salary – even if just for a while – may involve big adjustments to the life you're used to. Apart from less money coming in, you also have more expenditure. Raising a child is estimated to cost around £201,000 from birth to age 21. This equates to £9,610 a year, or £800 a month. Childcare is the single highest cost, amounting to an average of £54,696 per child from 6 months to 16 years.[17] I have friends who decided to get out of the rat race completely, downscale and move to a cheaper location. Studies continuously show that people who simplify their lives find the results to be overwhelmingly positive.

It can be tough adjusting to motherhood at first, especially if you're used to being independent and free. Looking after a child is hard work, and it never stops. You need patience, strong nerves and humungous amounts of positive outlook. Also you can feel very isolated and left out – a reason why mothers often form support groups. In the years I worked as a television foreign correspondent, I had to deal with high pressure, nit-picking editors and fickle interviewees. Nevertheless I have found motherhood to be the most demanding job I've ever done – and probably the most important. It has its monotony and thankless chores, admittedly, but it's highly rewarding in the long run. You're providing your child with a loving foundation for life; as the word 'sacrifice' suggests, you're giving a 'sacred gift'.

## HOW WILL A BABY AFFECT MY RELATIONSHIPS?

### Three for Company

Nothing will test your relationship with your partner quite like having a baby. The stress levels caused by a little mound of flesh demanding undivided attention 24/7 are enough to give Zen practitioners nervous twitches. Studies universally show that children take a major toll on relationships due to fatigue, less time spent together, less intimacy, more economic worries and more child-related disagreements and crises.[18]

> **'A baby is a hand grenade thrown into a marriage.'**
> NORA EPHRON, WRITER

A baby is a genetic mixture of yourself and whoever gave you his sperm. Having a child with someone means full-on commitment with a no-returns policy. If you truly want to be with this person, a child can deepen your love. It's the two of you morphed into a unique new human being.

Part of being a later mother implies that your relationship will hopefully be more stable to accommodate a third person. However, the whole reason you waited so long could be because you had yet to meet the daddy. Many friends of mine encountered their partners later in life and then got pregnant quite quickly with no time to waste. Having offspring was a real *getting to know you* experience.

The fathers of today are a new breed, more advanced in an evolutionary sense than our dads' generation. They no longer demand the *kid in bed and dinner on the table* by 7 p.m. You can find them on playgrounds holding sippy cups and wiping snotty noses, alone at parents' evenings because the wife is on a business trip, wearing aprons and cooking cakes for junior's first birthday party and patiently soothing temper tantrums. The average father today spends half an hour a day looking after his offspring[19] – that's triple the amount compared with a generation ago (or 30 minutes more than my dad looked after me).

## Friends and Happy Families

As for the other relationships in your life, expect a degree of transformation: bosom buddies may disappear into the wine-bar-post-work past and new pals will appear during park/playground afternoons (other people with young children, friendly tramps, etc.). Not everyone will share your interest in comparing baby wipes, or have the patience to keep repeating their sentences over an infant whining. If you value your childless friends, try and meet them alone and refrain from talking about the baby all the time. It pays to be sensitive to their situation; some of them may want cubs but just 'didn't get around to it'.

Producing kin can forge a new tie to your own parents. Dads are generally chuffed to be promoted to grandfather and your mum will adore being able to cuddle a bambino without the extra responsibility and being able to sleep through the night. Once you've given birth, the mother-daughter bond can become more meaningful. At the very least you'll appreciate what she went through to put you on the planet. However, there's also much new territory for strife. Your mama will have all sorts of tips on how to wean a baby/treat a cold/rear a child. It may have been the way to go in the 1970s, but fads change and there's been an enormous amount of research since then. The best you can do is bear with her; be tolerant, listen to her advice, say thanks and then do what you think best. Like all mothers she only means well (you'll recognize this behaviour in yourself the moment you're a mum), and let's face it: this is probably the only subject she feels she knows more about than you.

Not just mothers have useful/less advice you don't want to hear. Absolutely everyone will bully you with anecdotes about how their little lamb licked the loo brush, how to treat teething troubles, etc., from your work colleagues and siblings to a neighbour you've never met before (who doesn't even have children). The fact that you feel particularly vulnerable after childbirth doesn't help. Screaming at these people rarely improves matters. Practise a slow, understanding nod of the head instead; it will come in useful when your child reaches six and won't shut up.

As for other comments from the general public: if you're worried about whether the neighbours will disapprove of your bump or if the school gate mums will think you're the granny, say to yourself repeatedly, 'Who gives a shit?' Society is becoming more understanding with regards to delayed motherhood, but there are still some less tolerant members about. It's their problem, not yours.

## The Ultimate 'Are You Ready?' Test

1. Stay in every night of the week, even when you have the coolest invites to the hottest new venue in town. Every half hour or so, creep upstairs very quietly and peek through an opening of the bedroom door. If by the end of the week you still feel sane, congratulations; you've passed point 1.

2. Get someone to continuously thump or scrunch up the book/newspaper you're reading. If you can keep your cool, bravo. Proceed to point 3.

3. Try having a conversation with a friend over repeated cries of 'Mummy, Mummy'. Ideally you will have someone tug at your sleeve simultaneously. If you manage to finish your sentences and hear your friend out, without getting a headache, you're good to go to point 4.

4. Leave the house in the following manner: open the front door, shut the front door, open it again and, just when you've stepped out, go back inside! Then walk down the path, stop at a leaf, pick it up, turn it over and drop it. Look up and point. Then walk back towards the front door. Just before you get there, turn around and walk towards the garden gate. When you've reached it, repeat the same procedure you had with the front door. It's best to try this when you're running late for an appointment. If you can keep your nerve, go to 5.

5. Find or record a soundtrack of kids talking interspersed with baby crying noises. Play this on your iPod at full volume, and trying doing the following to it: drive your car/go clothes shopping/have a phone conversation/clean the kitchen/watch the news. If it doesn't bother you, try again with the volume turned up more.

6. Have a shower with the door open/curtain pulled back and one eye on the other side of the bathroom. Just when you're all lathered up, jump out and rush across to the other side (without slipping). Stay out of the shower in the cold for at least 2 minutes. Go back in and quickly wash off the soap, keeping one eye on the other side of the bathroom. Don't dry yourself off properly and put your clothes on as fast as you can. If you managed to clean yourself, you'll know you'll be able to shower with a baby.

7. Balance something heavy on your hip and try doing the following with just one hand: cook a three-course meal; put on make-up; write emails; go to the loo. Once you've successfully done those, try all of them again but add something clinging onto your leg. If you can manage without cheating, you're skilful and nearly ready to be a mum.

8.  Don't have spontaneous sex at any time during the test period. When you do have intercourse, pretend someone's barged in. If it's just before you're about to orgasm, that's realistic. Don't go back to sex (i.e. don't orgasm).

9.  Try having a meal (ideally a very nice one when you're particularly hungry) with a squealing, fidgeting animal on your lap – a baby piglet does a good job. If you manage to finish your meal without spilling most of it, then you can eat with a toddler.

10. Have someone wake you every three hours during the night and tug on your nipples until they hurt. At 7 a.m. get up, no matter how tired you feel. Repeat every night throughout the test period.

If you have successfully mastered all these points, you are theoretically ready to have a child – but be prepared for plenty more surprises when it's the real thing.

## THE COUNTDOWN

The healthier you are, the more fertile you'll be. I really can't accentuate this enough.

Good nutrition and a healthy lifestyle are even more important for later parents because they can make all the difference to your success at conceiving, carrying a healthy baby to term, recovering after birth and getting pregnant again if you choose to.

I would recommend every couple take a proactive approach and do a serious detox about 3 months before they start trying for a baby. As we age, our bodies have more accumulated toxins, so apart from hindering your chances of conception, these toxins will reach the foetus. Heavy metals, for example, pass over the placenta and can affect the baby's developing nervous system.

More and more evidence is emerging that the time in the womb shapes the rest of our lives. But it's not just the intrauterine environment of the mother that's important. Research in the new field of epigenetics has shown that DNA from the father will influence not just your child's health, but your grandchild's, too. It's highly advisable to stop smoking and cut down on alcohol at least 3 months before trying, because that's how long it takes for sperm to renew and the egg to ripen. Also cut back on coffee, processed foods and soft drinks and make sure you're eating plenty of wholefoods, fresh vegetables and fruit. Chapter 2 goes into plenty of detail on what foods are good for fertility and what to avoid. Most healthcare providers also recommend taking a folic acid supplement ahead of conception because it can help to prevent spina bifida.

This period of 'pre-conception care' is almost as important as the pregnancy period itself. Ideally prepare with not just a physical cleanse but a real emotional and mental purge as well: clean up old habits and make space for a new life. According to Ayurveda, human health has different layers, with spiritual health at the core. Spiritual health means living in harmony with your true purpose. It forms the basis of mental, emotional and physical health. A good diet, exercise, lifestyle changes and mindfulness can help bring a person back into balance so that pregnancy can really be an act of the whole body, spirit and soul.

# CHAPTER 2

## Keys to Conception: Enhancing Your Chances the Natural Way

### SEX, SEX, SEX

This would seem like a no-brainer: to get pregnant you need to have sex. But you'd be surprised how many people are not getting pregnant because they're not having ENOUGH sex. It's bizarre. We spend the majority of our lives doing the utmost to avoid pregnancy. Think about all that bonking you did when you were younger, and how petrified you were of getting pregnant. You spend years swallowing hormones, experimenting with flavoured condoms, squidgy sponges and dodgy pull-out methods. Then you grow up and only have sex when you're rested, the light is right, you haven't eaten too much or there's nothing on TV worth watching. And you expect to get pregnant like that. You basically need to have sex two to three times a week, spread out across the days (not twice on Sunday before and after brunch, although there's no harm in that either). The theory goes that the more nookie you're getting, the more you feel like it. But if that seems like too much effort and you want to target sex on your most fertile days, then read on.

## FERTILITY AWARENESS

Knowing when you are fertile can be as effective as the Pill if used properly. If you've never been pregnant before or have taken the Pill all your life, you have every right to be clueless as to when you're 'on heat'. This is your chance to get back in charge.

Basic biology dictates that for conception to take place, one fertile male sperm has to meet one fertile female egg. Sperm can survive inside the body for a maximum of six days, but the egg dies if not fertilized within 36 hours. So generally if you have sex a couple of days before ovulation until a day after, you're raising your chances of getting pregnant because it means the sperm are there waiting for the ripe egg. But when do you ovulate? This is where the arithmetic comes in and some women get a bit squeamish – so I'll warn you, this bit involves some sticky secretions.

Every month you have a small window of fertility – generally towards the middle of your menstrual cycle – when you ovulate. If you count the first day of your period as Day 1, then ovulation usually occurs around the middle of your cycle, generally between Days 11 and 16. There is no hard-and-fast rule, however, as every woman is unique and every month her cycle can differ, but it's useful to write down when you get your period so you start to get a feel for your menstrual rhythm.

Regular, pain-free periods with a good amount of blood are signs of a healthy cycle. The *rhythm method* by itself is not reliable enough to achieve pregnancy (or avoid it, as some randy teenagers may have found out) which is why you need to apply some other tricks.

'Having children is amazing but I'd say wait as long as you possibly can to have them. Then shag like crazy every day for a month and hope for the best.'

ADVICE GIVEN TO ME WHEN I WAS 28 BY A COLLEAGUE AT WORK; HE WAS 40 AND HIS WIFE 38 WHEN THEY BECAME PARENTS FOR THE FIRST TIME.

The key is noticing changes to your cervical secretions. 'Your secretions are your fertility,' points out the famous 'baby-maker', Zita West. By checking your underpants (yes, I said you might get squeamish) you can even predict ovulation. Highly fertile secretions look a bit like raw egg white. They are stretchy, slippery and transparent. Triggered by raised oestrogen levels, these bodily fluids indicate that ovulation is about to occur. It is also the best environment for sperm to survive and swim forwards in.

Shortly after ovulation your *basal body temperature* rises, which you can measure (with a lot of discipline). Secondary fertility signs such as soreness in the breasts or a slight pulling sensation in the abdomen, known as *Mittelschmerz*, can also give indications of ovulation taking place.

We don't necessarily ovulate every month, although research shows that ovulation can occur more than once a month.

There's no point, by the way, in using a fertility predictor kit if you're unaware of your cycle, because you could end up using it at the wrong time and think you're not even fertile. Predictor kits will only show when ovulation is about to happen. Cervical secretions begin a few days before ovulation.

### SUN AND MOON

Melatonin is a master control hormone that affects reproductive hormones and your cycle. Because the flow of melatonin is controlled by the blue component in natural white light, it's important to get as much natural light as possible during the daytime to stimulate your hormones. If you work in artificial light, go outside during breaks. Sunlight is also necessary for fertile egg and sperm, and vitamin D; so soak up the rays, especially in the British winter. Get rid of illuminated alarm clocks and electrical appliances in the bedroom, instead open the curtains on full-moon nights to regulate your cycle and boost fertility.

It's empowering understanding your fertility because it gets you more connected and in sync with your body. Apart from increasing your chances of getting pregnant, it can also make you a really bossy patient! My friend Carla was telling her gynaecologist her exact due date (later rather than earlier) because she knew precisely when she had conceived. It ended up in a minor disagreement, which my friend won, of course.

There's one snag to being in control of your fertility: sex can become mechanical. Intercourse timed with ovulation feels like a bit like a chore that needs to be accomplished while the dishes dry. Your partner will feel like he's on a stud farm (although that might actually turn him on, especially if you tell him he's hung like a horse). Hopefully he'll be able to deliver in what may be the most important performance of his life, although that pressure can be enough to send his friend into hibernation.

Many women do report that ovulation is the time in the month they feel most horny. A lot of female animals have more mojo when they're ovulating, sending the males crazy (ever had a dog?). So go for it, it's your primal instinct. Put on your caveman outfits and have some fun. What's hornier than shagging for a baby, anyway?

## How to Get Your Mojo Back

Eat libido-enhancing foods such as asparagus, oysters, truffles, celery, bananas, vanilla, cacao (every woman's favourite) and maca. Making a *Nine-and-a-half weeks*-style mess means it's had immediate effect!

> *'What I believe we must do as women is tap into our luscious fertility, have a sense of ourselves as sensual, sexual, fertile beings at any age. Honour your body, know when you're ovulating and understand the connection with the moon. We need to cultivate our receptive, feminine principles in life, our yin power as well as the deliberate pursuit of pleasure. Stop for afternoon tea and enjoy it, don't be in a mad rush to get everything done and check all your emails! Slow down and change your mindset!'*
>
> DR CHRISTIANE NORTHRUP

## TRUTH OR MYTH?

Have sex every other day if you're trying to get pregnant. Myth. Sex every day has been proven to increase chances.

Remaining lying down for at least 15 minutes after sex can increase your chances of getting pregnant. Truth. It helps sperm on their journey up the vagina and into the uterus. To avoid getting pregnant, the opposite would apply. Standing upright and vaginal showers will help wash the sperm out of the vagina.

Orgasm can help you get pregnant. Truth. Thanks to contractions sperm can be 'suctioned' up the vagina.

## FOOD FOR FERTILITY

It's official: the right food will boost your hormones and help you get pregnant. The wrong food can prevent you from conceiving.

Scientific research, extensive surveys and countless case studies all confirm it. It's what the fertility gurus up and down Harley Street and across the country are telling their reproductively challenged clients. Proper nutrition is vital for good health. The right diet is not only the key to fighting disease but it's also the answer to anti-ageing and improving and prolonging your fertility.

## Why Is Food So Important for Fertility?

The human body is a perfectly designed organism that has the remarkable ability to heal, rejuvenate and procreate. But for the body to work optimally it has to be in balance and the digestive system needs to be functioning well. If you're not eating the right food then the body is depleted and your hormones out of sync. Also, if you're ingesting too many toxins then a lot of the body's energy is spent eliminating them because the main aim is to regain balance. Reproduction won't be seen as a priority, because it isn't for immediate survival.

### THE POWER OF QI

In Traditional Chinese Medicine digestion is seen as key to vitality because it produces *Qi* (the Indians call this *Prana*) by absorbing nutrients from food. *Qi* is the flow of life energy. It's what surrounds us in the universe, keeps us alive and governs every function in our body.

For 30 per cent of cases of infertility, doctors cannot find an answer. But unfortunately most of them don't study nutrition at medical school. So despite all the scientific research linking nutrition to good health and increased fertility, couples are offered medication and expensive IVF treatments rather than being told to eat well (and, call me a cynic, but improving your diet doesn't make any money for the pharmaceutical industry).

## *What to Eat*

Food is basically your medicine and the far cheaper, less invasive option. Make sure you're eating enough vegetables and fruit: you need essential fatty acids (EFAs), omega-rich oils and antioxidants, and it's a good idea to eat a fair amount of your food uncooked. Organic food is best as it's pesticide-free and contains more nutrients. Local, seasonal produce is always to be preferred.

To ensure your body is absorbing nutrients you should cut down on (or cut out entirely if you can) ready-made meals and processed foods. Apart from having low nutritional value, they contain lots of hidden fats, sugars, salt and chemical preservatives which are toxic for the body. These foods also give you empty calories with short peaks of sugar levels, so your system won't be working optimally.

## *Fertility Foods*

Try to include plenty of the following in your diet for improved fertility. These particular vitamins, minerals and EFAs balance the reproductive hormones and protect against DNA and chromosomal damage.

### Vitamins

| | |
|---|---|
| **Vitamin A** | alfalfa, apricot, asparagus, broccoli, cabbage, carrot, garlic, kale, papaya, peach, pumpkin and pumpkin seeds, spinach, sweet potato, tomato, turnip, watercress |
| **B Vitamins** | alfalfa, algae, almonds, asparagus, avocado, banana, beetroot, brewer's yeast, broccoli, cabbage, kelp, lentils, mushrooms, nori, spinach, sunflower seeds, walnuts |

| Folic Acid | avocado, brewer's yeast, broccoli, brown rice, cauliflower, dates, leafy greens, lentils, oats, orange, spinach, wholegrains★ |
| Vitamin C | alfalfa, apple, apricot, asparagus, avocado, beetroot, bell pepper, blackberries, blueberries, cabbage, citrus fruit, kiwi, onion, papaya, strawberries, watercress |
| Vitamin E | alfalfa, almonds, brown rice, blueberries, leafy greens, nuts, sesame seeds, sunflower seeds, sweet potato, wheatgerm |

## Minerals

| Calcium | alfalfa, almonds, broccoli, oats, cabbage, leafy greens, spinach, sesame seeds |
| Iron | alfalfa, almonds, apricot, avocado, beetroot, brewer's yeast, chickpeas, dates, figs, kidney beans, leafy greens, lentils, parsley, pear, pumpkin, raisins, spinach, sunflower seeds, watercress |
| Magnesium | alfalfa, apple, apricot, avocado, banana, brewer's yeast, brown rice, cacao, celery, fig, grapefruit, leafy greens, molasses, peach, sesame seeds, sunflower seeds, wholegrains★ |
| Manganese | alfalfa, avocado, blueberries, chickpeas, leafy greens especially spinach, lentils, pineapple, sunflower seeds, wholegrains★ |
| Selenium | alfalfa, avocado, brazil nuts, brewer's yeast, broccoli, brown rice, garlic, onion, parsley, sesame seeds, spinach, sunflower seeds, wholegrains★ |
| Zinc | alfalfa, almonds, asparagus, avocado, brewer's yeast, carrot, leafy greens, oats, pecan nuts, pumpkin seeds, sunflower seeds, sea vegetables, shellfish such as oysters, sweetcorn, tomato |

★Wholegrains include amaranth, barley, buckwheat, corn, millet, oats, quinoa, rye and wholegrain rice

## Essential Fatty Acids

Get vital omega 3 from linseed/flaxseed oil; hemp, perilla, krill or chia seed oil.

Omega 3 (DHA) is also found in oily fish such as sardines, mackerel and salmon (beware though: some fish oils, such as cod liver, can be contaminated).

Vegan DHA supplements are derived from marine micro algae.

Evening Primrose Oil helps produce more fertile cervical fluid; but take it only from menstruation to ovulation as it can provoke contractions.

> *'Essential fatty acids are really important for fertility because they keep the egg cell membranes healthy and soft for sperm to penetrate more easily. Trans-fats are bad because they make the outside of the egg harder.'*
>
> DR MARILYN GLENVILLE

## Superfoods

Bee pollen is the ideal fertility food because it's the seed of the plant kingdom. One spoonful is packed with amino acids and proteins that are easily absorbed by the body.

Royal jelly is a fertility superfood said to increase egg quality and even quantities. It's the only food a queen bee eats – and she lays 2,000 eggs a day. If you're allergic to bee stings, you shouldn't eat bee pollen or royal jelly.

Chlorella is a chlorophyll-rich algae that helps the body remove heavy metals, dioxins and pesticides and repair DNA. It's also rich in $B_{12}$, and is alkaline and blood-building. Take a supplement or spoonful daily, two hours before or after meals.

Maca is THE fertility food of the Andes. A nutrient-rich root that grows high up in the mountains, maca helps balance the endocrine system and hormones. I add a spoon of maca powder to my breakfast smoothie daily.

## Herbs

Use Agnus Castus or Wild Chasteberry, Black Cohosh, Dong Quai and False Unicorn Root. These herbs can all effectively balance hormones and regulate periods to increase fertility. Remember herbs are quite powerful and shouldn't be taken if you are on any other medication or hormonal treatment.

## A Word about Supplements

Much of today's fruit and vegetables are nutrient-deficient because the soil has become so depleted; this is why nutritionists often advise taking supplements. However, if your body is out of balance it won't absorb the nutrients from supplements well either. Eating a plant-based diet of organic wholefoods is the best basis you can have. You can add sprouts, algae and oils to ensure you're getting more concentrated forms of nutrients. If you're adding a multivitamin in tablet form make sure it's the best you can afford (100 per cent wholefood rather than synthetic) and check for your specific needs.

> When diet is wrong medicine is of no use.
> When diet is correct medicine is of no need.
> — *Ayurvedic Proverb*

## *Why Choose Organic?*

Studies repeatedly show that organic foods have more nutrients with higher-quality vitamin and mineral content and more antioxidants than non-organic foods.[1] Organic food tastes better and is also free of the pesticides that are making our soil and our populations barren. Many of the pesticides used today contain *xenoestrogens*. These chemicals mimic our natural oestrogens, confusing the body's hormone receptors and creating infertility.

Here's some compelling evidence: conventional farmers and men employed in agriculture or pesticide-related jobs are ten times more likely to suffer from infertility. They were shown to have a significantly lower proportion of normally shaped sperm.[2] The sperm count of organic farmers showed up a super potent 363m/ml with very little abnormal sperm[3] (compare that to today's average sperm count of a meagre 60m/ml).

If for financial or logistical reasons you can't get organic produce, peel any fruits you suspect to be heavily sprayed (apples, for example), and soak berries, grapes and green leafy vegetables for several minutes in water with some lemon juice, apple cider vinegar or food-grade hydrogen peroxide before rinsing. Thick-skinned fruit such as watermelon, pineapple, banana, avocado and papaya are not as susceptible to damage.

If you have a local farmers' market, shop for your groceries there. Talk to the farmers, because often even if they don't have the organic label – which is costly and legally complicated – it may be that they're not using pesticides (and hopefully no genetically modified organisms [GMOs] either). It's better to eat fresh, local food than organic produce that was picked two weeks ago and flown in from South America.

## Raw Revolution

It's a fact of modern living that mass animal food production is destroying our planet. Intensive livestock farming for meat and dairy puts a strain on the environment because it requires so much energy and water. It takes 200 times more water to produce a pound of beef than a pound of potatoes, and livestock eat 70 per cent of the world's grain. Lowering your meat consumption – or even going vegetarian – means you're reducing your carbon footprint. Aside from this political, environmental agenda, eating a vegetable-based diet – at least 50 per cent raw – has overwhelming health benefits. We're actually the only animal that voluntarily cooks its food before consuming it. A baby calf, for example, will not grow into a strong adult cow and may perish if fed its mother's milk in pasteurized rather than raw form

When food is cooked above 45 degrees the molecular structure of enzymes is broken down and destroyed. You can see this by watching any vegetable lose its colour and elasticity when you cook it to death. Raw, *living* food has a higher vitamin and mineral quality and intact enzymes. These enzymes help us digest food and remove old, diseased tissues from the body. Enzymes are also responsible for DNA repair and organ healing. If your body has to draw on its own source of enzymes to complete the job of digesting food, it basically ages more rapidly. Our organs cannot keep up with eliminating waste, and this accumulation leads to an overall toxic state in the body, causing illness. Enzymes are literally the spark of life.

Another way to explain the raw food concept is through energy. High-resonance foods can convert and carry more energy into the cells of the body, increasing your subtle electrical energy field. Research indicates that nutrition with a frequency over 72MHz increases the body's electrical energy. Foods below this drain the body's power reserve (processed foods barely reach 10 to 30 MHz).

By introducing more raw food into your diet, you will notice your mind and body feeling clearer, clean and vibrant. Try making a fruit smoothie for breakfast, have a green smoothie mid-morning, then have a big salad followed by some sprouted beans, grains and seeds for lunch. If it's cold, as it often is in Britain, you can end the meal with a soup and make a warm, nourishing protein-rich meal for dinner. Or start by introducing a raw food day once a week. When you do cook, remember to steam or grill rather than boil or fry, to preserve more of the food's nutritional value and avoid those evil trans-fats. If you remember to eat raw food before cooked food you'll strengthen your immune system and counteract leukocystosis, which is basically the body recognizing the polypeptides from cooked food as foreign invaders.

## SPROUTING

By growing your own sprouts you have one of the cheapest and most powerful ways to supplement your diet. Sprouts are literally bursting with vitamins, minerals, proteins and huge amounts of enzymes. Sprouts are a less expensive and far superior protein source to meat. You just need some seeds, a plate or jar, water and within 2 days to a week you can increase the nutritional content of any seed a thousandfold. Try sprouting watercress, alfalfa, chickpeas, lentils and sunflower seeds.

## BEATING THE CLOCK

Biological age and chronological age don't necessarily have to overlap. By following the previous nutritional advice you can help your DNA repair itself. By increasing your intake of antioxidants and protecting your cells from toxins you can combat ageing and prolong your fertility. You can also boost your growth hormones – the key to anti-ageing and elevating sex hormones – by fasting or detoxing.

## Oxygen, Water and Salt

Apart from the right food, plenty of oxygen and adequate hydration are vital to good health. Many of us are not breathing properly and living in polluted cities, so we are generally oxygen-deficient. Going for regular walks in the countryside or in a park (if you live in a city), breathing deeply and practising yoga, qi gong or tai chi will oxygenate your blood.

Dehydration is a relatively easy problem to solve – you basically need to make sure you're drinking enough water, which is at least two litres a day. Any diuretic substances like black tea, coffee, fizzy drinks or alcohol will dehydrate your body, so you need to compensate them. Cellular damage, rapid ageing and disease can be the results of not drinking enough water. Hydration is important for good follicles and a strong blood supply to the womb. Most of us are dehydrated and we don't even realize it because having a dry mouth is actually the last sign of dehydration. From 1983 until his death in 2004, the Iranian Dr Fereydoon Batmanghelidj impressed the scientific community with his powerful evidence illustrating that many diseases, including cancer, are caused by unintentional dehydration. His simple WaterCure is a cheap and very effective treatment. To find out more, take a look at www.WaterCure.com.

The best time to drink water is 30 minutes before meals and 2 hours after food so that it doesn't interfere with the digestive juices. Another way to make sure your body is absorbing water is by adding a pinch of real salt – but not the white poison on the tables of most restaurants and on the shelves of the supermarkets, which has been stripped of all minerals through chemical processing. Himalayan crystal salt or unprocessed sea salt contains over 82 essential trace minerals. Ancient healers knew that salt is one of the treasures of our planet. It's found in most of the water on earth and inside rocks and mountains, and in our blood and the fluid surrounding our cells; our bodies are in fact 70 to 80 per cent saline. The amniotic fluid in the womb has a similar salt consistency to that of the ocean – babies basically swim in salt water for the first 9 months before birth.

## Long-term Advantages

If it seems too difficult to change your eating habits radically, you can start slowly and build up. As you introduce more healthy meals, you'll feel the difference and start craving wholefoods. However, it's not worth obsessing about because being too strict isn't healthy, either. Sugar is one of the hardest addictions to give up but luckily there are now alternatives. If you've never tried raw cake sweetened naturally with xylitol, coconut or agave syrup, you'll be amazed how good it tastes.

Taking a proactive approach means you're optimizing your chances of carrying a healthy baby to term. Pregnancy and birth can deplete you, so eating well will help you bounce back quicker after birth. This is especially important when you're older and hoping to have more children. As a later parent you probably want to be fit and healthy as long as possible anyway. All the tips apply to your partner as well, because nutrition affects his health and fertility, too. And just wait until your baby starts eating solids: you'll care about what goes into her unfinished, sensitive digestive system.

## DETOXING

### Toxic Overload

Detoxing has become something of a buzzword in recent years, but this is definitely a case where you *can* believe the hype. We live in a toxic environment and no matter how careful we are we can't avoid toxins because we eat them, breathe them in and absorb them through our skin. Moving to a remote island to live in a bamboo hut is not a realistic option, but we can massively cut down on the toxins we're absorbing through food, cosmetics and the products we use around the house.

The shelves of supermarkets (or 'stupormarkets' as some like to call them) are crammed full of mass-produced, processed foods. By consuming these products we're ingesting large amounts of chemical preservatives, additives, sugar, hormones, antibiotics and other barren-makers. But there is some good news here: a) you can choose to buy more organic, wholefoods and b) you can get rid of toxins by cleansing regularly (at least once or twice a year). Detoxing is a great way for maintaining good health and has also been proven to give growth hormones – the anti-ageing angels – a huge boost.

Anyone trying for a baby later in life has a very good reason to detox because as we grow older, poisons accumulate in our bodies. By the time we've reached our late thirties and early forties the toxins may have built up so much that they're clogging up the cells, sending the hormones out of balance and preventing conception. A good fast will get rid of the toxic overload and acidity in your body. Even for those who conceive easily, it's a good idea to detox a couple of months before getting pregnant because it will clean out your intestines, improve food absorption and make you stronger for pregnancy, birth and breastfeeding. Toxins and heavy metals in the mother's body will pass over to the foetus so it's highly recommended to go on a fast a few months before you hope to conceive. A detox will also make you review what you put in your temple of a bod, so it can be a great way to revolutionize your eating habits.

Due to our Western diet of too much white flour, processed bread, fizzy drinks, meat, dairy and fast food most of us have unhealthily high acidity rates. Disease thrives in an acidic body but not in an alkaline environment; detoxing can help neutralize the acidity. A body that is alkaline also produces the right cervical fluid and sperm.

Common symptoms resulting from accumulated toxins are headaches, bad breath, allergy symptoms, PMS, fatigue, depression, irritability, bloating, constipation and frequent infections. A hair analysis or kinesiology screening can determine your toxin levels and draw relevant detox recommendations. You could also do a blood test to check for allergies.

## Fasting and Detoxing

Detoxing is very simple but it's important to get some guidance if you've never done it before. You can do simple juice fasts and juice feasts at home where you basically make yourself various juices throughout the day; some fruit, others veg. Not only are you cleaning your system but you're also loading up with nutrients. There are also a wide range of detox supplements and herbs you can take if you're cleansing from the top down i.e. without colonics. Some of them contain oxygen to liquidize the compacted faecal matter; others have psyllium, which absorbs toxins. Toxins are released via the colon, liver, kidneys, skin and lymphatic system, so it's a good idea to support a detox with massages such as MLD (Manual Lymphatic Drainage). You need to ease in and out of fasts by eating a vegetable-based diet, preferably as uncooked as you can. If you want to undertake a longer or more radical detox, seek advice from a nutritionist. There are many good places to fast around the world and this can be a great pre-conception holiday.

A study on detoxing showed that after a one-week green juice fast with a supplement of liquid zeolite, 88 per cent of participants had eliminated 100 per cent of all toxins and heavy metals in their bodies. Those who continued for a second week showed a 100 per cent reduction of all toxins and heavy metals. More proof of the body's remarkable ability to heal.[4]

Don't do a detox if you're already pregnant, as the released toxins will pass into your womb. If you're worried about having too many toxins you can adjust your diet to incorporate more vegetables and fruit, especially in the first half of the day. This will clean your body in a more gentle way. Remember that your insides are very clean and virginal after a detox, so it's even more important what you eat and drink immediately afterwards.

### EASY LIVER CLEANSE

Drink a cup of warm water with the juice of lemon first thing in the morning, especially if you drink coffee. Lemon and orange juice help restore the alkaline balance in the body and neutralize the effects of acidic coffee.

## Toxins to Avoid

Often people will want to part with hard-earned cash to be told by someone in a designer suit to cut back on the unhealthy snacks and bad habits. I'm giving you the list here, for free (or included in the price of the book). The only difference is I won't be checking up on you. Show this list to your partner, because it all applies to him as well. If he needs more proof, the section on *fertility for him* (page 53) should provide some answers.

Cut back on:

- *Non-organic meat* – contains antibiotics and hormones that interfere with the reproductive system
- *Non-organic animal products* such as cow's milk, cheese and eggs – contain antibiotics and hormones
- *Processed food and ready-made meals* – chemical preservatives, hidden fats, sugars and bad salt
- *Low-fat foods* – chemical additives and low nutritional value
- *Low-fat dairy products* – many more water-soluble hormones than full-fat versions
- *Chemical flavourings* such as MSG (mono-sodium glutamate or 'flavour-enhancer' found for example in most soya sauces) – shown to cause infertility when tested on animals[5]
- *Trans-fats* (hydrogenated fats often added to products to increase shelflife, processed cooking oils) – just 4 grams of trans-fat daily – found in one doughnut or a plate of chips – can double the infertility risk[6]
- *Soya foods* – shown to contain oestrogen-mimicking properties; small amounts of soya in its fermented form such as miso and tempeh, are fine.[7]
- *Aspartame* (artificial sweetener in diet sodas, chewing gum and sugar substitutes) – accumulates in cells, causing damage to DNA[8]

- *Soft drinks* – two or more of these a day lead to a 50 per cent greater chance of ovulatory infertility.[9]
- *Cosmetic products* – look out for preservatives in face cream, formaldehyde in nail polish and aluminium in deodorant, check labels and try to buy products without chemicals.[10]
- *Amalgam fillings* – proven to release dangerous quantities of mercury vapour on a constant basis; if you can have them replaced with white, ceramic ones.[11]
- *Pharmaceutical drugs* such as antibiotics, antidepressants, antihistamines, anti-malaria pills, antivirals, decongestants, inhalers, sleeping pills, painkillers and steroids
- *PFCs* (common industrial perfluorinated chemicals used in Teflon, waterproof clothing, food packaging, upholstery and pesticides) – interfere with the reproductive hormones and are known to stay in the body for decades. A study showed that exposure levels seen in the general population can reduce fecundity.[12]
- *Soft plastics and cellophane* – contain oestrogenic chemicals that can leak. Never drink bottled water that has been allowed to heat up in the car.
- *Aluminium* (pans, tin foil, kettles) – a heavy metal that is toxic in the body; replace cookware for glass, enamel, stainless steel and earthenware.[13]
- *Unfiltered tap water* can contain chemicals from detergents and hormones.
- *Household detergents and cleaning products* – many of these contain APEs (alkylphenol ethoxylates) which mimic oestrogen and cause reduced sperm count.[14] Use natural alternatives: white wine vinegar, lemon juice and baking soda.
- *The big three*: **smoking, alcohol and caffeine**[15] (see below)

You may ask why all these products are legal if they're so bad for you. The products are subjected to little Government testing and even then they're checked in isolation, so 'safe' is a very relative term. We mustn't forget the power of corporate lobbies and the oil industry (from which many of these products are derivatives) and their entanglement with the authorities. For these barren-makers to disappear from the shelves, consumers have to stop buying them.

Remember to chew properly and don't eat too fast. Avoid eating if you're stressed, upset or angry, as this produces more toxins. Overeating is another cause of toxicity, so try to eat up to 80 per cent of your capacity. Gosh, don't I get the good job? (Believe me, I'm genuinely *not* a bossy person!)

### LENTILS FOR BEEF

A famous Harvard study involving 18,555 nurses showed that the women who ate more red meat were the most likely to have ovulation problems leading to infertility.[16] It is a fallacy to believe that we need to eat meat for our nutrients. An average serving of quinoa has more protein than a steak, and a handful of sesame seeds or a spoonful of tahini are a better calcium source than a glass of cow's milk. Humans, unlike carnivores, have very long intestines where ingested meat rots and we don't produce the special enzymes needed to neutralize the uric acid in meat. Hence numerous studies also show that vegetarians and vegans have a better pH balance and far fewer toxins in their bodies than those who eat meat.

## Smoking

When we grew up, puffing was cool. Marlboro cowboys were still riding into the sunset and sexy women everywhere smoked. But the proof has finally been laid on the table and plastered across cigarette packets. Smoking is detrimental to health and it's also to blame for infertility. It literally poisons the ovaries. It doubles the free-radicals in the body and increases the intake of lead, cadmium and other additives, which are toxic to cells. By smoking you're robbing your body of oxygen and the antioxidants important for fertility such as vitamin C and selenium. If an egg does get fertilized it's less likely to implant; miscarriage rates for smokers are much higher. Women who smoke are twice as likely to be infertile as those who don't and it can even bring on early menopause. But the good news is if you stop smoking, so do the negative effects on fertility.

Another reason to quit smoking for good is that scientists now believe that DNA damage is epigenetic – which means the expression of the DNA is carried from one generation to the next. So, apart from all the other known problems such as under-weight, pre-term babies, a smoking mother is seriously damaging the DNA of her offspring. Men whose mothers smoked during pregnancy were even shown to have decreased sperm counts of up to 40 per cent.

## Alcohol

Here comes the next party-spoiler. Alcohol is a big no-go for when you're trying to get pregnant (and when you are pregnant, but more of that later). Alcohol has been proven to reduce fertility by half. The more your drink, the less likely it is that you will conceive. Cutting down to fewer than 5 units a week (that's about five small glasses of wine) will double your conception chances. Or better still, cut out alcohol altogether if you can. It's a serious culprit of cell mutation.

Research shows that there's a 70 per cent increase in sensitivity to toxins, alcohol and smoke on the day preceding ovulation. This would include secondary smoke, so try to stay out of smoky environments during this part of your cycle. If you're going to have a drink, indulge in a really good glass of wine during your period and dilute with plenty of water.

## Caffeine

Drinking as little as one cup of coffee a day can halve your chances of conceiving. Caffeine consumption is also linked to increased chance of a miscarriage. Caffeine comes in many disguises: coffee in all its shapes and forms from latte to espresso, the British classic builder's tea, coke and other fizzy drinks, energy drinks and, sorry to say, ladies, but chocolate, too. However, cacao in its raw form is said to improve fertility. If you've never tried raw chocolate, this is your chance – it tastes like the real thing because it *is* the real thing.

It's not a tragedy if you drink the odd coffee, but if you drink a coffee, a tea, a coke *and* eat a bar of chocolate all in one day, you've exceeded the dose that is seen as healthy for conception and pregnancy.

## Can't Be Bothered?

This may all seem like a huge sacrifice to make. If you have a lifestyle that involves a lot of stress, drinking coffee to keep you going and alcohol to relax, it's going to be hard to change your habits. We live in a culture where binge-drinking is more normal than juicing. If you don't join in the inebriated party, you can be seen as a freak. But this is about you getting pregnant. Think about it as paving the way for your future child. Wouldn't you rather be holding your dream baby than an empty glass?

## DE-STRESSING

Now if all this talk about toxins has got you worried and I tell you not to get stressed about it, how do you feel? Better? Of course not! The last thing you want to hear when you're stressed is, 'Just chill out.' It's like all those people saying, 'Just relax and then you'll get pregnant.' Yeah, right! But, unfortunately, it has been proven that too much stress can lower your chances of conception. It's all about the hormones. Hormones are the nuts and bolts of baby-making.

## *Why Is Stress Bad for Reproduction?*

As all stockbrokers know, stress produces adrenalin, the fight-or-flight hormone. But what may be doing it for a 23-year-old wanting to avoid family at all costs, definitely isn't working for a 40-year-old seeking to procreate. Adrenalin has an adverse effect on hormone balance and it can block progesterone, which is vital for a pregnancy to implant successfully in the womb. It can also upset the pituitary gland which is instrumental in preparing for ovulation and conception. Other hormones released by stress are cortisol, an important one for the balance of hormones in the body; and prolactin, which can interfere with regular ovulation. Reducing the stresses of modern life will regulate the hormones needed for reproduction.

### SCIENTIFIC EVIDENCE

A study of 2,000 couples suffering from infertility showed that stress was the main cause in 25 per cent of cases.[17] Another study of women who had been struggling with infertility for more than three years found that 44 per cent got pregnant within 6 months after taking part in a stress-management mind–body programme.[18]

## *Neutralizing Stress*

Breathe in deeply, count to ten, breathe out slowly, count to ten, breathe in … etc.! Shallow, short, irregular breathing reflects that we're under stress (and most of us are more stressed than we think). When we're relaxed, breathing becomes calm, deep and regular. Correct breathing is one of the best ways to manage stress. If you've ever watched a newborn baby sleeping, you'll be astounded how deeply they breathe. It's because they haven't started copying adults yet, who've mostly lost that ability.

Techniques like yoga, qi gong and meditation are so popular these days because we're encouraged to use the breath in a nurturing way, bringing us back to our origins. It also means we're pumping our lungs full of oxygen. No wonder you come out of class feeling high.

## QUICK DE-STRESS EXERCISE

Sit down for 5 minutes and breathe warm pink light into your belly. Visualize it flowing all over your body.

There are many measures you can take to combat stress; the obvious one being to take a break. A holiday can be a wonderful way to forget about your daily grind. But it's no good if you come back refreshed and are forced straight back into an exhausting rut. If you're unhappy with the ways things are, find out if you can make some adjustments. Maybe you can share your workload, reduce your hours or work from home a day or two a week. Less time spent on trains/buses/cars and in an airless office environment can greatly improve the quality of your life. If you're stressed because you're home alone with a young child, then practical things like getting help cleaning (if you can afford it) can be a godsend; so can sharing childminding with other mothers, in order to get some time off to yourself.

My father (who's still voluntarily working at 67 and unlikely to retire anytime soon) always says there's negative stress and positive stress. Positive stress is healthy because you're enjoying what you're doing. Whereas negative stress – the cancer culprit – makes you sick because you're doing something you don't enjoy. So the key is feeling more positive about your work, enjoying the parts of it you're particularly good at and focusing on that. If none of this is possible, maybe you should think seriously about changing jobs or taking a very long sabbatical.

On your free evenings and weekends, do the things you REALLY enjoy. Indulge and nurture yourself, even this means sitting in front of the TV with a tub of your favourite ice-cream. Take long baths using aromatherapy oils; listen to music with headphones; go to bed early with a book. A good night's sleep is so important for mental wellbeing. Try and do some active things too, preferably in nature, as this is very healing and energizing.

### SPACE-CLEARING

Make sure your bedroom doesn't have stagnant energy, as this can interrupt sleep and block fertile energy. De-clutter and remove any TVs, stereos or computers so there's no electro-magnetic pollution. Take anything you don't need or love from the room. You can perform a space-clearing ritual simply by using intention. Think of creating a sacred and safe space for the hours you rest.

Massages and bodywork are worth indulging in. Apart from relaxing tense muscles, these treatments work on a deeper level, bringing your physical and mental body into alignment. If you can't afford treatments take a free, local massage course and team up with other participants to work on each other. Or see if you can do an exchange with any therapist friends you might have. A massage for an hour's accounting or gardening for example.

On top of the stress of daily life, you may be stressed out trying for a baby, especially if it's taking longer than you had hoped. Hypnotherapy is great for addressing subconscious anxiety (see the section on complementary therapies, page 51).

Research on infertile women showed 80 per cent of them resumed ovulation after 20 weeks of psychotherapy to reduce stress levels.[19] Simple self-applied acupressure, such as meridian tapping and EFT (Emotional Freedom Technique) are thought to speed up psychotherapy by balancing the disrupted meridian energy system (Qi or Chi). The method proved to eliminate stress response and regulate ovulation in just a few sessions (more details follow in the next section).

## FIT FOR FERTILITY

We live in a society focused on image. It's all about looking beautiful, young and sexy. There's a strong culture of external exercise and the gym has become an intrinsic part of modern culture. Sports like aerobics, weight-training and running may tone your muscles, make your body look great and increase your stamina, but they're not doing much for your internal body. Yoga, tai chi and qi gong are all ancient arts that were conceived to massage your internal organs and calm the mind; exercise from the inside out, so to speak. Also, because they're not vigorous or high impact, they're ideal for boosting your fertility and you can continue all of them throughout pregnancy.

Most of us are too static in our lives; we sit at desks (rather than reach and twist to pick apples off trees, as we were designed to do), so it's important to find some kind of balance. Yoga, tai chi and qi gong are shown to increase circulation to the uterus and ovaries. They also strengthen the endocrine and reproductive systems. Different postures can help direct blood to the sacral area of your body to augment your conception chances. Imagine drawing warm, pulsating energy towards your sexual organs and womb while you flow through the movements.

### GIVE YOURSELF THERAPY

Meridian tapping or EFT is a good way to free up blocked emotions and damage caused by difficult or traumatic experiences. It allows you to tackle stress issues at their source, and energy imbalance as well as unresolved negative emotions. It's also a great way to get energy flowing through the body to increase fertility. You basically tap along the meridians in your body and focus on specific emotional issues you'd like unblocked. The energy points are the same ones as used in acupuncture and you can easily teach yourself the method (free downloads are available off the internet).You can also learn how to give yourself fertility massages. Gently massaging your uterus and ovaries will remove stagnant blood and increase the flow of fresh, oxygen-rich blood to the area.

When you're doing yoga, it's a good idea to vary your practice (or the intention of your practice if you're attending classes) according to the phase of your menstrual cycle. In the first weeks your focus could be to nourish and grow strong, fertile eggs; direct attention to your ovaries and think about producing abundant cervical fluid. In the days preceding ovulation your practice can be more energetic and all about releasing potential. Then in the last part of your cycle, where implantation occurs or your period comes, try to feel more at one with your yin energy, which is the power of waiting, being open and receptive. This is also a time to rest more and nurture yourself.

## FOCUSING THE MIND

### Think Positive

Similar to when they proved the world was round rather than flat, quantum physics has revolutionized what is actually possible. We now know that everything is vibrating, from the book you're reading to the surface you're sitting on. Quantum physics also proves that you ARE your thoughts and that your consciousness affects what's around you and, interestingly, ahead of you. So all that 1980s talk about positive thinking was not so far off; you do actually have the ability to manifest your dreams.

According to a phenomenon called the Law of Attraction, all things in the universe that vibrate at the same frequency are attracted to each other. In other words, like attracts like. This means that what you think and feel will be attracted into your life. Energy flows where attention goes. So if, for example, you're constantly thinking, 'Why am I still not getting pregnant?' or 'Everyone has a baby but me,' you're focusing on the problem; this will attract more problems such as infertility and lack of pregnancy. Compare, for example, the snowball effect of a bad day when everything seems to go wrong, or how you get increasingly angry during an argument.

To change the situation you need to get out of negative thought and energy patterns. Exchange destructive mindsets or feelings like 'I don't deserve this' for new, more joyful ones. By focusing your attention on good things, your body and cells will receive more positive messages. Thoughts like, 'I will get pregnant when the time is right' and, 'I will become a mother' are more likely to attract what you so much desire. Once the thoughts are vibrating on a positive level, your feelings and emotions should also follow. As they say, *Change your thoughts and you change your destiny.* The final step is to let go of expectations and trust in the process. Learning how to meditate can be useful, if you find this hard.

> *'Repeating a statement about something being true will create neural connections as though we were experiencing the thing being true and were making a statement of fact.'*
>
> DAVID HAMILTON, *HOW YOUR MIND CAN HEAL YOUR BODY*

## Affirming and Visualizing

Thoughts are seeds that become reality. If you believe a thought, the body follows because every cell in the body is influenced by the mind. Based on this insight you can practise simple techniques to get mind and body connected. Affirmations and positive visualizations will send messages to your body that it's fertile and strong enough to conceive and carry a pregnancy to term. Affirmations can be very simple, such as the yogic one: *Sat Nam*, which translates as 'The truth is my identity.' Or you can make up your own affirmations: 'I am a magnet for good things,' 'I am secure enough to let go.' You might want to try conception-focused ones such as 'My ovary is releasing a ripe egg, I trust that I will get pregnant when it is meant to be and I am in perfect health to become a mother.' Performing a fertility ritual – which can be as simple as lighting a candle and making a wish – is also a good way to attract what you want into your life.

> 'A woman told me we should send out a cosmic wish. We went to the Seychelles on holiday and sat under the stars holding hands, both wishing very strongly. We did a ritual to ask for a child to come to us. I know I got pregnant on that day because I also did an ovulation test.'
>
> MECHTHILD, BABY AT 43

Visualization works along similar lines. Picture yourself enjoying perfect health while you silently repeat the affirmations. Visualize ripe follicles, a plump endometrium and a fertilized egg bursting with life, making its way down your Fallopian tube. Every morning before you get up, visualize there's already a baby in your belly, and recapture this feeling various times in the day. If these are too specific for you, visualize white light entering your body from the crown and, as it spreads down through your body, allow it to heal every organ. Alternatively you can picture nourishing energy seeping up from roots below you in the earth, giving you strength and fertility. A Tibetan Buddhist technique is to breathe sunlight into your heart centre and then ground it by growing roots into the earth. By meditating like this regularly you can even 'clean out' damaged cells and heal bad cellular memories.

## Accepting What Is

As disappointing as it may be when you get *yet another period*, keep staying positive (am I beginning to sound like a self-help coach here?). See it as a chance for your body to get even stronger and healthier for the next time. You might think it would be better to get pregnant in February so your baby is born early November and it's all calmed down in time for Christmas (just as an example), but this is one thing we really can't plan. In the grand scheme of things your pregnancy will come at the right time because life is – in its own funny way – perfect. Everything is exactly as it is meant to be. Once you learn to trust this concept, you'll be able to let go, be receptive and embrace what comes your way with less resistance.

## COMPLEMENTARY THERAPIES

A good plan of action for getting pregnant may include complementary medicine. Apart from helping you relax, therapies such as acupuncture and reflexology work on the energy systems to aid the body to heal itself. Acupuncture has gained recognition for helping balance hormones and regulating periods. Hypnotherapy has very good results with couples who have unexplained fertility (which could be stress-related.) In this section I will only cover a few techniques. It is also worth looking into aromatherapy, homeopathy, Reiki, Bowen, vibrational healing, massage and various others to enhance fertility. A course of treatments will add up, but it's still a lot cheaper than IVF.

### Acupuncture

Acupuncture has its origins in the East, where it still plays a big part in daily healthcare. Traditional Chinese Medicine (TCM) is around 5,000 years old and views each patient as his or her own universe. TCM and TJM (Traditional Japanese Medicine) believe that disease implies an imbalance within the body. Health is determined by a harmonious flow of vital life energy, known as Qi (also Chi or Ki). Qi travels along 14 major pathways, called meridians and when stimulated these have the power to heal. Bad diet, stress or viruses can obstruct Qi, resulting in disease.

Another way to explain how acupuncture works is through electricity. We are a bit like mini-generators. If you were able to 'plug in' your body it would produce more electricity than is needed for a whole house. Imagine the body like a giant powerhouse of electrolytes whose purpose it is to bathe the cells in an electrically active fluid. All reactions that occur in the cells are electrical in nature.

> *'The doctor of the future will give no medicine, but will interest his patients in the care of the human frame, in diet, and in the cause and prevention of disease.'*
> THOMAS EDISON (1847–1931), INVENTOR OF THE PHONOGRAPH, LONG-LASTING LIGHT-BULB AND MOTION PICTURE CAMERA

## Ayurveda

Ayurveda comes from India – based on spiritual texts called the Vedas – and is also around 5,000 years old. Ayurveda believes that everyone is made of different combinations of the five basic elements in the universe: space, air, water, fire, and earth. Poor nutrition and stress can throw you off-balance, resulting in illness. Treatment involves a series of restorative processes such as cleansing and detoxification, herbs, meditation, massage and other lifestyle modifications to restore physical, mental and spiritual health.

> *'There's a difference between biological age and chronological age; with a healthy lifestyle your biological age can remain youthful even if you're over 40.'*
> DR GOWRI MOTHA

## *Hypnotherapy*

Hypnotherapy has been known to help cases of infertility where no physical cause is found. It's very effective if you have problems letting go because it produces deep states of physical and mental relaxation. Hypnosis is naturally induced and allows suggestions to be communicated to your subconscious mind – the part that influences how you think, feel and choose. You can be taught the deep breathing technique of self-hypnosis, or a therapist can guide you to a relaxed state where your subconscious is activated. Therapists also provide counselling. You may have some underlying issues holding you back, such as a difficult relationship with your mother, childhood trauma or other experiences in the past. There could be subconscious fears at play – like fear of giving birth or fear of caring for an infant – which are getting in the way of a successful pregnancy.

One method is to focus on an objective such as getting pregnant. Hypnotherapy can also be used to distract you from what has become an obsessive focus of attention, such as getting pregnant. They are simple measures that can resolve deep emotional blocks.

## *Reflexology*

By stimulating specific reflex points in the foot that correspond to organs and parts of the body, healing can take place and balance re-established. Reflexology has been known to help with cases of infertility by balancing and reducing stress in the body. It has also had good results in maintaining the pregnancies of women who suffered from recurrent miscarriage.

## FERTILITY FOR HIM

New studies suggest that fertility is becoming more of a man's than a woman's problem. But most gynaecologists focus purely on the girl, not because she's prettier, but because that's what they're trained in – female reproduction. A good GP or fertility specialist should check you *both* out.

## Sperm Crisis

Environmental toxins, synthetic water additives and hormonal substances in food are all blamed for the dramatic deterioration of male sperm over the past decades. The average sperm count in the 1940s was 100 million sperm per millimetre of semen (m/ml). That was before the introduction of grand-scale industrial farming using pesticides. Today the average sperm count is around 60m/ml. In the United States – a country that loves its junk food – the sperm count decreased[20] as much as 50 per cent from 1982 to 1992. The number of men with low sperm counts has tripled in the Western world over the last decades, and it seems to be getting worse. A particularly shocking recent study showed that 20 per cent of men between the ages of 18 and 25 (those potent years) have drastically abnormal sperm counts of less than 20m/ml; this is defined as functionally sterile.[21] The number of men with reduced sperm motility over the last decades has also increased, from 21 per cent to 43 per cent – that's nearly half the male population.

New research shows that sperm quality also decreases with age. Out of 12,000 couples treated at a fertility clinic in Paris, it was found that women whose partners were 35 or older had more miscarriages than those with younger men, regardless of their own age. Embryologists blamed the miscarriages on genetic defects in the sperm, which build up with age. If there is too much DNA damage, the body's natural repair mechanisms are overwhelmed. Embryos with serious DNA damage are spontaneously miscarried. Other research shows a slight increase in birth defects in babies born to older men.

So that's the depressing stuff. You can see we're all in the same boat; the worldwide fertility crisis is affecting young and old alike.

The good news is that you have the possibility to change it. Your hubby/boyfriend/designated father of your child can do a lot to improve the quality of his sperm. By eating the right foods and cutting back on alcohol, smoking, drugs and coffee he can get his sperm fit. Remember, new sperm are produced every 100 days, so he needs to kick any bad habits 3 months prior to conception.

## *What to Cut Out*

### Smoking
Decreases sperm count, makes them more sluggish and increases the number of abnormal sperm. Smoking inhibits zinc absorption – a vital mineral for male fertility – and it depletes the antioxidant functions of vitamins leading to DNA damage in cells. Paternal smoking has been shown to increase the risk of childhood cancer in your future baby by 70 per cent.

### Drinking Alcohol
Decreases sperm count and motility and increases the amount of abnormal sperm. It also inhibits zinc absorption and interferes with testosterone production. It has been found that 80 per cent of alcoholics are proven sterile because alcohol is a testicular toxin. A binge drinking weekend will still be affecting sperm 2 months later; however, sperm return to normal after 3 months if alcohol is given up.

### Coffee
Cut out or cut back on coffee. Research shows that the problems with sperm increase with the number of cups of coffee consumed daily. Coffee, black tea and alcohol also dehydrate the body. Hydration is very important in order to create a good environment for sperm movement. A dehydrated man can have what's known as 'clumped sperm' – not good.

### Anabolic Steroids

Steer clear of any anabolic steroids; they upset the hormonal balance in the body.

### Stress

Stress doesn't have such a great effect on men, either. Research has shown that stressful situations such as a death in the family or separation cause temporary abnormality in sperm. The good news is that the sperm do recover when the stressful time ends.

### Tight Underpants

Tight underpants (honest!) and hot baths are linked to poor sperm quality.

### Mobile Phones

Radiation from mobile phones is also blamed for infertility issues in men; keep phones out of trouser pockets and turned off when possible.

### Toxic Substances

Water-soluble paints, paint strippers and glycol ethers lead to sperm abnormality. Men regularly exposed to these substances, such as builders and decorators, were found to be 250 per cent more likely to have problems with fertility.

Pesticides and hormones in non-organic foods are detrimental to sperm and testicles.

The toxins and the guidelines mentioned in the *Detoxing* section (page 36) also apply to men.

## *What to Include*

Eat fresh wholefoods rather than refined, processed foods. Follow all the nutrition advice mentioned in the *Food for Fertility* section (page 28). In order to produce good, strong sperm, men need sufficient B vitamins, vitamin C, vitamin E, selenium and zinc. Zinc is found in high concentrations in sperm and is needed to make the outer layer and tail. If there is one supplement to take for sperm, it would be zinc.

Additionally men need to make sure they are getting the amino acid L-arginine, which is found in the head of the sperm, by eating plenty of nuts, oats and a spoonful of bee pollen for breakfast.

Your future baby receives 50 per cent of its DNA from the father. If you can encourage your fella to work with you on this, it is a good exercise in shared responsibility; and there'll be plenty more of that later once the baby comes along.

## THE MIRACLE OF CONCEPTION

This is a little story about an egg called Erin and a sperm called Sebastian.

When Erin – our egg in this story – was born, there were 2 million potentials just like her. She belonged to the tiny minority who would reach maturity. Each month, one of her sisters was released from the follicle, until the time came for Erin to ripen. It took her 90 days to get ready for ovulation. She was thrust on her journey into the Fallopian tube and knew she had only 24 hours, so she started sending out signals to attract her Mr Right.

Sebastian – our sperm – was only six weeks old when he was released alongside 300 million brothers into the vagina. Sebastian swam forward as fast as he could and made it with 1 million others to the cervix. The signals and scents being sent out by his destiny were so strong he was able to reach the Fallopian tube in half an hour. The distance was 2,000 times his length, or around 3 km (17 cm in human terms). Alas, 200 suitors just like him had also made it; as a prize, all their heads were fortified by special enzymes from the liquid inside the Fallopian tube.

Sebastian waited a while, maybe it was even a day. All of a sudden, he felt her presence; she was covered in that thick, soft protective coating called the *zona pellucida*. She was irresistible. He immediately recognized that the molecules on her surface were meant for him, and this led him to swim in a hyperactive, staccato fashion. Erin also recognized his molecules and pulled him closer. Most of his brothers bounced off her thick skin, but Sebastian was healthy and strong enough to penetrate through a small tunnel he burrowed. He was the chosen one.

Erin immediately went through massive chemical changes; her cell membrane shut out all other sperm and she bundled half of her genes (23 out of 46) and pushed them out. Once firmly implanted inside her, Sebastian lost his tail and rested. A few hours later he was a changed sperm; his head had grown and he was ready to meld his 23 genes with Erin's remaining 23 inside her nucleus. The membranes between their cells dissolved and their chromosomes doubled. They were creating a new organism. This first cell would be the blueprint for the future adult body's 10 trillion cells. The miracle had occurred.

# CHAPTER 3

## Pregnant with a Little Help from Modern Science

### WHY CAN'T WE GET PREGNANT?

*Panic Stations*

If you're used to getting what you want in life by effort, perseverance and sheer hard work, then not being successful at getting pregnant can make you feel betrayed by your own body. But before panicking and calling the IVF clinic, you have lots of options to explore first.

Infertility is known to affect one in six couples in the UK at some point in their lives, although the latest research indicates this figure is increasing to 25 per cent. In the US, one-third of women over 35 are believed to have fertility problems. Statistics suggest it takes the average couple about 8 months to get pregnant naturally. Or, put differently: 80 per cent conceive within a year. People are generally told to get checked out if they've been trying for a year or two without success. However, women over 35 will be aware of the pressure – both from their surroundings and from themselves

– to 'not waste too much time'. A 39-year-old friend of mine in New York was told by her doctor that if she didn't get pregnant naturally within 3 months she would be put on fertility drugs. This ludicrous suggestion, involving pretty serious drugs, is just another example of how couples trying for a baby aren't being supported in the right way. There is a huge boom in IVF, with many couples being directed towards expensive medical treatments when these are not actually necessary. An acquaintance told me confidently that most of her friends were having IVF and that she had booked her first appointment. After asking a few questions I realized this woman had no idea about the fertile phase of her cycle or how she could improve her chances of conception.

There are many reasons for sub-fertility, divided more or less equally between male and female factors. Sometimes there's more than one problem; you may suffer from endometriosis and your partner may have a low sperm count, for example. Other reasons could be vaginal infections such as candida, hormonal imbalances or ovarian cysts. The most common cause of infertility – one-third of all cases – is 'unexplained'; this means doctors can't establish any specific medical problem. This is where you have to delve a little deeper for the answer – it may be related to lifestyle factors, nutritional deficiencies or emotional/psychological elements.

No one will care as much about your fertility as you do, so avoid handing over the responsibility to a doctor or clinic. You can find a lot of answers in this book; it really isn't complicated. It simply involves both partners making the effort to get as healthy as possible – so basically you can only gain from the process. You have a very good chance of carrying a baby to term when your body is ready. Also don't forget the mental and spiritual aspects of conception; being calm and balanced will make you much more receptive.

## Correct Diagnosis

First you need to examine if your lifestyle is preventing pregnancy or causing miscarriage. Are you having enough sex? Are you drinking a lot of coffee to keep you awake, and/or wine to help you wind down? Are you dehydrated? Are either of you binge-drinking? Are you living off fizzy or diet drinks and grabbing food on the go? Often slight changes can make a big difference, so follow all the advice in Chapter 2.

Get a hair analysis to check for toxins and deficiencies, and follow it up with the relevant detox. You can simultaneously have a health check for STDs or other medical problems that may be causing infertility. If after this you're still none the wiser, it's worth putting together a plan of action and maybe working together with a professional – be that a GP, fertility expert or specialist in complementary medicine.

A good specialist will investigate both male and female fertility issues. They'll look at the possible medical reasons but also factors such as diet, lifestyle, work and exercise. If failing to conceive is of a medical nature then it's still worth checking out various solutions. Don't feel pressurized into taking what appears at first to be the easy way. Drugs have side effects and surgery takes time to recover from, and can result in complications; so in the end it could be the longer route. Supporting your body to heal itself is a more solid foundation for a successful pregnancy.

*'I was told I'd never have children because of the massive damage to my body and internal organs from being shot when I was 17. But I have a daughter, who is 33 now. I'd say listen to the diagnosis but don't believe the prognosis. Focus on being healthy, vital, and strong in every aspect rather than focusing on the problem.'*

DENISE LINN, AUTHOR AND SOUL COACH

In many cases Western medicine can be effective, but the disadvantage is that it tends to take a *one size fits all* approach. By seeing a GP or specialist who takes an integrated approach – combining Western and complementary medicine – you'll find a solution that is more individually tailored to your needs and specific issue. The most successful fertility specialists all recommend trying the complementary route first or combining it with medical treatment, if this is genuinely needed. This integrated approach is the way the future of healthcare is moving.

> *'Many women I see have had hard knocks from the medical profession. When you're older the anxiety levels are higher because of all the statistics and the press who give older women a hard time. But there are many things you can do yourself to improve fertility. A correct diet will improve the environment the egg is growing in, whereas smoking and alcohol damage every cell in the body. You can also support the environment; acupuncture helps increase blood flow, so the nutrients get to the ovaries. It's about changing your mindset, too. Women want to feel supported and have a good plan of action.'*
>
> ZITA WEST, FERTILITY EXPERT

Holistic care can prepare you physically and mentally for conception. Numerous studies have now shown that acupuncture improves fertility,[1] as it balances reproductive hormones and helps strengthen blood, which is important to nourish and sustain a fertilized egg. If there are psychological issues preventing pregnancy then hypnotherapy and healings such as family constellation work have shown to be successful.

## Options Checklist
1.   Diet and lifestyle adjustments

2.  Course in complementary medicine

3.  Medical therapy such as fertility drugs

4.  Reproductive surgery

5.  Assisted conception such as IVF

## *False Hopes*

Another reason why I'm so adamant about trying everything possible first is that, according to the available statistics, the success rate for fertility treatment goes down dramatically with age. At the moment the so-called *take home baby* rate is around 10 per cent for women doing IVF between 40 and 42 years of age; in some clinics it is even as low as 2 per cent. Doctors say it's because of the decrease in egg quality. But often it's because couples are not correctly informed on what they can do themselves to improve the outcome of IVF.

> 'We spent 8,000 Euros on IVF because the fertility clinic said we'd never get pregnant naturally with my partner's sperm. The drugs made me feel really sick, I would never have survived the pregnancy. Anyway the IVF did fail and I became very disillusioned with the production-line practice of the clinic. After that experience, we waited a while, my partner stopped smoking and 2 months later I got pregnant naturally. IVF is all about making money. Just don't let them rush you into it.'
>
> MARTA, BABY AT 43

Many fertility clinics in the UK won't perform IVF on women over 42 because they say the odds of a live birth are too low. Clinics all want to be at the top of the league table, so by excluding older patients they're aiming to enhance their success rates. It also means that the IVF success rates for older women won't improve. Many women turn to IVF as a last resort after a long history of being 'sub-fertile'. A conclusive IVF study of healthy women over 40 doesn't exist, for obvious reasons.

> A study showed that 80 per cent of couples with a history of infertility got pregnant naturally after following a pre-conception care programme involving changes in diet and lifestyle.[2] This success rate is FOUR times higher than that of the best IVF clinic.

## GETTING TESTED

As a UK citizen you're eligible for basic fertility investigations on the NHS at your GP's surgery or a sexual health clinic. Being over 35 means you have the right to be referred straight to a specialist. You should be asked about your medical history and given a physical examination. You might have to do a smear test and have a scan. Urine and blood samples are taken to check for chlamydia or any other sexually transmitted disease (STD). A survey at a Foresight clinic showed two out of three clients suffered from genito-urinary infections, also known as STDs. These diseases can go unrecognized for years and be a major cause of infertility. Blood tests are also taken to check for immunity to German measles and your hormone profile. Your partner (or designated sperm donor) would also be tested for STDs, and he will need to give a sperm sample to check for abnormalities. It makes sense to have all these tests done on the NHS, because a private fertility clinic is more likely to get you straight onto the IVF route.

You can do other tests independently, such as the hair analysis I mentioned earlier, which will tell you what vitamin and mineral deficiencies or heavy metal excesses you have. A simple hormone test requiring saliva samples across the month measures oestrogen and progesterone levels, and gives an indication of problems with ovulation or progesterone levels.

## *All About the Eggs*

Some clinics will offer the test for egg reserve but, despite the hype, this test is really not that reliable. All it does it measure the baseline level of follicle-stimulating hormone (FSH) on Day 3 of your cycle, which can give an indication of how close to the menopause you are. It won't tell you exactly how many eggs you have left; it can just give you an idea whether your so-called *ovarian reserve* is average for your age. This result is thus not particularly conclusive, unless you differ a lot from the norm. The test cannot say anything about the *quality* of the eggs you have left, either. You may, for example, have a low ovarian reserve but eggs that are of good quality, which would mean your chances of getting pregnant are pretty good.

> Researchers removed stem cells in the adult mouse ovary and implanted them into the ovaries of sterile mice. These then formed new eggs, and the mice gave birth to healthy pups.[3] This remarkable finding challenges the belief that females are born with a set number of oocytes and suggests that old ovaries have the potential to produce new eggs.

Egg freezing has received a lot of attention recently due to numerous babies successfully being born from frozen eggs (rather than frozen embryos as is the case in IVF treatments). Because this technique is still rather new and experimental, it's not really an option for later mothers today. However, as the vitrification technique improves, it does mean that young, single women can freeze their eggs for use, say, 10 or even 20 years later. As a consequence, the number of later mothers is bound to keep rising.

A US study on IVF compared two donor egg groups (age 21 to 30/age 31 to 40) and found pregnancy outcomes to be similarly successful.[4] So may we question the notion that fertility decreases with age and assume that 'older eggs are just as good'?

## Choosing a Clinic

The NHS covers the costs of some fertility treatments, such as IVF, although at the moment if you are over 39 you have to fund your own treatment as a private patient. Private fertility clinics set their own prices, and what's included differs from clinic to clinic. Some clinics offer so-called 'treatment packages' which include basic consultations, scans, tests and treatment procedures. Asking for a personalized, costed treatment plan will give you a better idea of the final amount you'll be expected to pay. Fertility drugs are usually charged extra, and these are rather pricey. Some clinics cater to specific treatments or age groups, so find one that suits you. Also, if during any part of your treatment you feel your clinic is not doing you justice, then you should go somewhere else.

The Human Fertilisation and Embryology Authority (HFEA) regulate clinics in the UK, so if you choose to go abroad for fertility treatment, you should be aware that clinics will adhere to different codes of practice. The EU Tissues and Cells Directives also set out quality and safety standards, but not all countries in the EU/EEA have implemented the legislation.

At any UK fertility clinic you and your partner will need to sign consent forms for the use of your sperm, eggs and embryos. Free counselling is available at many clinics and is worth taking, as the waiting and hoping can be physically, mentally and emotionally wearing.

## Sticking Together

Sub-fertility can be a great strain on a relationship. It's hard to be patient with your partner if you've given up drinking and he hasn't, for example. Keep communicating and try not to blame one another. There may be a lot of underlying resentment or guilt at hand. Women generally like to talk more about conception issues, to the point where it becomes excessive for the man, who prefers to go over things just once or twice. Don't be afraid to seek support in getting through this as a couple. And don't forget your sense of humour; some of the concepts in fertility treatment are so abstract and clinical that the best thing you can do is have a laugh about it together.

## MEDICAL THERAPY

For healthy ovulation an egg has to be produced and released each month. So-called 'ovulation dysfunction' can be a consequence of hormonal imbalance, blocked Fallopian tubes, fibroids or an ovarian cyst. You may have irregular or painful periods as a result. Most women don't ovulate every single cycle, and it seems that, as we approach the menopause, we ovulate less frequently. Having said that, some theories hold that women ovulate *more* as they age because the body is giving fertility one last shot.

The first step in medical therapy is fertility drugs – such as Clomid – which help trigger egg production. Most hormonal drugs are taken orally. There are also treatment cycle drugs used to regulate menstruation; these are usually injected. The main disadvantage is that, as with most pharmaceuticals, there can be side effects. Hot flushes, headaches, mood swings and nausea are some of the common complaints. Also Clomid, which is used to induce ovulation, has the downside of thinning the uterine lining, making it harder for an embryo to implant. It's therefore not suitable for women who have been diagnosed as blood- or yin-deficient by an acupuncturist. Other risks of taking fertility drugs are ovarian hyper-stimulation syndrome, ectopic pregnancy and multiple births.

Women undergoing IVF treatment will be given a course of fertility drugs in order to overstimulate the ovaries to produce more eggs for collection.

It depends on how severe the problem is, but a lot of ovarian dysfunction can be treated with complementary medicine. You'd need to have regular treatments over about 3 months to see results, although success can be achieved much faster than this.

## REPRODUCTIVE SURGERY

More serious cases of blocked Fallopian tubes, ovarian cysts, fibroids or endometriosis can be treated by *keyhole surgery* or *minimally invasive surgery*. Other names for it are *laparoscopic* or *endoscopic surgery*. Operations are performed through small incisions in the tummy button and close to the pubic hair line. A tiny camera relays images which are then magnified onto a TV monitor to aid the operation. It usually requires a general anaesthetic.

Sometimes conventional surgery is performed, which requires a 10-cm long bikini-line cut.

Reproductive surgery is performed on men who cannot produce sperm due to an earlier vasectomy. Sterilization can sometimes be reversed or, if it can't, sperm can be retrieved for use in fertility treatment.

The risks with these treatments are minimal but, as with any operation, there are the usual disadvantages such as your reaction to anaesthetic, and recovery time. Remember you need time to build up your blood after surgery, so this has to be calculated in before you start trying to get pregnant.

Cysts and fibroids should be monitored but often they disappear without medical intervention. I was diagnosed with a 2.5-cm cyst on my right ovary. The doctor said we should check it in a few months but that I probably needed surgery to remove a cyst that size. I detoxed, had a few sessions of acupuncture and breathed healing light into the area during meditations. I also visualized healthy ovaries and sincerely believed I didn't have a cyst. The next scan, 4 months later, showed the cyst had gone.

## INTRAUTERINE INSEMINATION

Intrauterine insemination (IUI) involves 'washing' semen in a laboratory to separate fast-moving from slow or non-mobile sperm. The fast sperm are then inserted, via a small catheter, into the woman's uterus during the time of ovulation. An IUI can be given with or without fertility drugs. It can also be performed using donor sperm. The whole process takes a few minutes and is usually quite painless, aside from maybe menstrual-like cramping.

The procedure is usually offered to couples with mildly abnormal semen analyses or those wanting to use donor sperm. IUI is generally used if there is unexplained infertility or if you have ovulation problems. If IUI is unsuccessful then IVF is often recommended.

### WORTH THE HASSLE?

Researchers in Scotland monitoring 580 couples found that common fertility treatments such as Clomid and IUI had absolutely no benefit. The success rate with drugs was even lower than those who were told to 'just go home and get on with it'.[5]

### Sperm Donors

All HFEA-approved sperm donors in the UK are interviewed, screened for diseases and offered counselling. Donors are paid for expenses and loss of earnings, but financial compensation is minimal so that this doesn't become a motivating factor. The HFEA say two out of three sperm donors are over 30, and 41 per cent of them already have children. In the UK a donor has no legal responsibility or rights towards the child conceived using the donation but the child can, when she is 18 years of age, find out who the donor was. It is seen as a criminal offence for internet sperm companies to procure or distribute sperm without a licence from the HFEA. Practices differ abroad so it's worth finding out the clinic's screening and recruitment process, if you choose this option.

'I went into the fertility clinic wanting to freeze my eggs and came out with an IVF plan using donor sperm. They told me I was literally on my last follicles. What gave me confidence was when the pretty young receptionist said, "My colleague and I decided not to take any donors we wouldn't want to use ourselves."'

KAREN, TWINS AT 42

## GAMETE INTRA-FALLOPIAN TRANSFER (GIFT)

GIFT is a semi-invasive procedure where eggs are removed, mixed with the man's sperm and inserted via catheter into the Fallopian tubes. This relatively new technique allows fertilization to take place inside the woman's body, so conception occurs close to naturally. Only the healthiest eggs and sperm are selected, thus increasing the chances of pregnancy. The Fallopian tubes have to be open and healthy for the procedure to work. Eggs are removed from the ovaries using *keyhole surgery* which involves a 5-mm cut at the belly button. Demand for GIFT is low and only a number of UK clinics are licensed to offer it. It's usually offered to patients who have failed IVF attempts, so success rates tend to reflect this.

## IN-VITRO FERTILIZATION (IVF)

As far as fertility treatments go, IVF heralded a brave new world for assisted conception when the first so-called 'test tube baby', Louise Brown, was born in 1978 in Oldham. Since that day, IVF has become a routine procedure – but it is expensive. Most people still pay for their own treatment, costing between £4,000 and £8,000 per round.

For many women and men with a history of infertility, IVF is a chance to have their own genetic child. It means the baby can grow inside the mother's womb and be born naturally. It also allows gay couples to have children and single women to become mothers by using donor sperm.

*In-vitro* fertilization literally means fertilization 'in glass'. Treatment can vary from clinic to clinic, but a typical procedure would involve the following:

1. Your monthly hormone cycle is suppressed using a daily injection or nasal spray.
2. Your egg supply is boosted with a fertility hormone or FSH (Follicle Stimulating Hormone) for 2–4 weeks. FSH increases the number of eggs you produce so that the clinic can fertilize more eggs and have a bigger choice of embryos to use.
3. Ultrasound scans and blood tests are used to monitor your progress and you are given a hormone injection to mature the eggs 34–38 hours before they are collected.
4. The eggs are collected from each ovary via ultrasound and a needle. You are sedated, but cramping and some vaginal bleeding can occur after the procedure.
5. Over the next few days you take pessaries, gel or injections to help prepare the lining of the womb for embryo transfer.
6. The eggs are mixed together with the sperm in a culture dish in the lab for about 16–20 hours. Those that have been fertilized

– the embryos – are grown in the laboratory incubator for a couple of days.

7. The best one or two embryos are chosen for transfer for women under 40. If you are over 40, maximum three can be used. Good remaining embryos can be frozen for future attempts. Some clinics also offer IVF at a reduced rate if you donate eggs to others (egg sharing).

8. Then you have to wait ... If the embryo implants in your womb and continues growing, soon pregnancy symptoms may start appearing. Two weeks after transfer you can do a pregnancy test.

## Improving Your Chances of IVF Success

### Preparation

Getting yourself ready for IVF is something to be taken very seriously. It can massively boost your chances if you are physically, mentally and spiritually prepared. Ideally you'll have followed the diet and lifestyle advice in Chapter 2; this includes giving up smoking and drinking alcohol. Remember, IVF can't improve the quality of your eggs, only you can do that. Eat lots of greens to support the liver and make sure you're getting enough essential fatty acids (through oily fish, flax/hemp seed oils or a daily DHA supplement). You also need to up your intake of vitamin C, vitamin E and selenium because these antioxidants will help neutralize the free radicals the liver produces, when it deals with the toxins of IVF drugs. You can drink dandelion tea to decongest the liver and start the day with a glass of hot water with some squeezed lemon. You also need to strengthen your blood supply beforehand – this is important to counterbalance the effects of the drugs and build up the uterus lining. Drink nettle tea for the blood and eat lots of iron-rich foods such as beetroot, spinach, oatmeal, lentils, kidney beans and watercress. Snack on seeds, almonds soaked overnight in water, figs, dates and raisins. Make yourself a green juice with chlorella powder daily; you can alternate by adding spirulina. If you can, stop drinking black tea – the tannins can prevent minerals from being absorbed. Your IVF unit may encourage you to drink more milk for its protein, but many people today don't tolerate lactose well. You could try milk in its fermented form as yoghurt or eat lots of sprouts and quinoa.

It's proven that stress is very counterproductive to IVF; one study showed that being anxious about missed work, money or medical intervention increased the IVF failure rate[6] by 30 per cent. The procedures are very cold, medical and clinical, so it's important to breathe some humanity into the process. On a mental–spiritual level it would be good to prepare by meditating, resting and focusing your intention on providing a warm, nurturing home for the embryo. You can also try affirmations, meridian tapping and visualizations using a warm colour such as orange.

## During the Treatment

IVF is minor surgery so you need to support your body to heal well after egg retrieval, in order to be ready to receive and nourish the embryo. Take the homeopathic remedy arnica the day before IVF starts; vitamin C, vitamin E and zinc also help wound healing. Rest well and drink more water than you usually do. If you can, take a few days off work when the embryo is transferred and enjoy lie-ins and early nights. Exercise only gently: no high-impact sports but do continue walking, doing yoga, tai chi or qi gong. It's important to keep your belly and womb warm at all times for the embryo to implant successfully. So if it's cold wear extra layers around your middle and sleep with a hot-water bottle.

As for the mental–spiritual aspect, 'communicating' with the embryo can play a decisive role. An IVF mother is under much more stress and pressure to succeed than a mother who conceives naturally. During natural conception there is a constant hormonal dialogue between cells during the journey down the Fallopian tube. Once arrived in the womb the new embryo then also makes its presence known to the mother by releasing hormones. In IVF, the fertilized embryo is transferred into the womb rather suddenly. It helps if you can mentally prepare a home for your embryo and then visualize your cells growing together after transfer. Send love and warmth to your embryo to convert the energy of the medical instruments it's been exposed to. This dialogue can be very subtle, just an intention is enough. Be receptive, welcoming and nurture the fragile life-form which could grow into your child. Keep the womb connected to the heart and practise being loving towards yourself and your surroundings.

> *'The main problem with IVF is implantation. Most women reach embryo transfer and the embryos can be good but her body doesn't take the pregnancy. If that problem could be tackled the live birth rate would be much higher.'*
>
> DR MAGDY ASAAD, DIRECTOR LONDON FERTILITY CENTRE, SPIRE HEALTHCARE

Apart from being relaxing, a course of treatments in acupuncture, reflexology, massage or hypnotherapy can be very supportive of IVF. Complementary therapy can help to prepare, detox and balance the body, grow follicles and build up the womb lining, support implantation and maintain the pregnancy.

## For Him

If your partner can also follow the advice in Chapter 2 to improve his sperm, you have better chances of IVF working. This means stopping smoking and drinking 3 months prior to treatment, and improving his diet. The more damaged his DNA the lower the chances of a healthy embryo and the higher the miscarriage risk.

During treatment your partner can support you by helping you stay calm and rested. He can also 'welcome' the future child and spend time placing his hands on your womb to keep it warm and protected. The IVF procedure for men is generally simple. Your partner will be asked to produce a fresh sperm sample which is then washed and spun at a high speed in order to retrieve the most active sperm. Donated sperm is removed from frozen storage and prepared in the same way.

### GENTLE IVF

Cutting out the harsh effects of medication is now possible by having 'soft' IVF, which uses minimal doses of drugs and 'natural cycle' IVF where no drugs at all are used. Both options are considerably cheaper and less disruptive to the woman's body. A Dutch study even showed much higher success rates and experts believe an older woman responds better when her ovaries aren't overstimulated.

## Expansions of IVF

IVM (In vitro maturation) is a technique where the still immature eggs are removed from the ovaries and then matured in the lab before being fertilized by the sperm. It basically means that you don't have to take as many drugs before the eggs are collected.

Another variation of IVF is ICSI (Intra-cytoplasmic sperm injection) which involves injecting a single sperm directly into an egg in order to fertilize it. This allows IVF to take place even if there is a very low sperm count or previous attempts failed due to a low fertilization rate. It can also be used if your partner has had a vasectomy and sperm have been collected from the testicles.

And now for another long, medical term: pre-implantation genetic diagnosis (PGD or, also, PGS) is used to avoid the risk of transmitting an inherited disease by examining the chromosomes in the embryo before implantation. It is often offered to those suffering from infertility or recurrent miscarriage due to chromosomal issues, because only healthy embryos are transferred to the womb. This form of genetic testing is also used for sex selection, although it's illegal to use it for this purpose in the UK. It appears that PGD increases the chances of pregnancy – but it adds to the cost of IVF.

## Egg Donation

If IVF is failing due to the quality of your eggs, then it's possible to use a donor egg. Because the age of the uterus is practically irrelevant this option is interesting for much older women. If you're suffering from early menopause or have low FSH levels you have the chance to get pregnant, carry a baby to term in your womb and give birth by using a donor egg. A donor can even be someone in your own family, such as a younger sister or cousin. Egg donation is advised if you have numerous failed IVF attempts due to poor egg quality. Waiting lists for donor eggs are long.

## Assisted Conception Health Risks

The greatest health risk associated with assisted conception is multiple births. Being pregnant with twins (or even triplets) can mean health complications for the mother and babies. The babies are more likely to be premature and have below-normal birth weight. If you want to avoid a multiple pregnancy you can ask your clinic to use single embryo transfer. This means you're less likely to have twins but also decreases your chances of getting pregnant. Other risks are bad reactions to drugs, especially ovarian hyper-stimulation which is an overreaction to fertility drugs. Ectopic pregnancy – when an embryo implants outside the uterus – is also more common in women having IVF, as are pregnancy

PREGNANT WITH A LITTLE HELP FROM MODERN SCIENCE

complications involving the placenta and vaginal bleeding. Fertility treatments are known to lead to more health risks for the children; IVF babies have higher rates of autism, cancer and other disorders such as cerebral palsy.

## SURROGACY

Surrogacy is where another woman carries a baby for you. Even though it's a legal minefield it can be the only option if you can't medically undergo pregnancy. This could be due to an absent womb or womb malformation, recurrent miscarriage or repeated IVF failure. There are two types of surrogacy: partial and full surrogacy. Partial or traditional surrogacy is usually performed by IUI. Your partner's or chosen father's sperm are injected into the uterus of the surrogate mother in order for fertilization to take place with one of her eggs. The surrogate is therefore both the genetic and the carrying mother. During full or host surrogacy the surrogate receives embryos that are not genetically hers. It can be embryos created from your eggs and your chosen sperm transferred to her womb. Or she can have IVF with an embryo created by a donor egg and your chosen sperm or the third option is IVF using both donor egg and donor sperm. The odds are similar to any assisted conception treatment. There is a risk of transferring HIV and hepatitis, so everyone involved is screened.

### *Home or Abroad?*

It's recommended to get legal advice before you go ahead with surrogacy because the laws are complicated and you'll want to be recognized as the legal parent. The fertility clinic won't be able to find a surrogate for you because the HFEA doesn't regulate surrogacy. Commercial surrogacy is illegal in the UK, so you're not allowed to pay a host mother anything more than expenses. Agencies offering such services, beyond the law, exist but there are also free networks and surrogacy support groups. When choosing a surrogate it's worth building up a relationship with her and trusting she will have a healthy, safe pregnancy.

With long waiting lists in the UK, the pull to go abroad where laws are more lax is increasing. Couples may go to a country such as India to seek a surrogate mother. This *womb for rent* phenomenon is a controversial subject. There is little regulation and it's becoming a multi-million dollar business. Cynically labelled the *globalization of reproduction* or *pregnancy outsourcing*, there are of course numerous ethical concerns. Are the surrogate and donor women being exploited or is it an opportunity of empowerment for them, as they can make a substantial amount of money? How will the child feel about it? Regardless of the difficult issues, it is giving hope to infertile couples worldwide.

'I had my womb removed due to ovarian cancer when I was 34 and nearly died from surgery complications. Living without a womb made me feel like I wasn't a real woman and I abandoned the idea of ever having children. I was often depressed and had nightmares of my ovaries being thrown into a bin. One day my partner brought up the subject of family and it churned up lots of emotions. I was too old for adoption in Switzerland, so we decided to try surrogacy. After some research we went to India and found a clinic we liked. My partner gave them a sperm sample and we chose a surrogate but she didn't show up at the last minute. After months we picked a new woman and this time treatment went ahead. We were sent photos of the two embryos before implantation. I was mesmerized and fell in love with them immediately. I bought a book and followed the foetal development day by day. But after 2 months we found out the embryos had stopped growing. The clinic offered to try again but I couldn't have gone through the procedure another time. It took a while to heal and symbolically let go of the unborn children in my life. I realized I can be a mother in other ways, and have become a magnet for the children of family and friends.'

KIRSTEN, 45

## ADOPTION

Adoption brings together a child who needs a parent and a parent who needs a child. The connection to an adoptive child is just as profound as to your own genetic offspring and in many cases people have spoken of spiritual or past-life links. There is no upper age limit for adoption in the UK, but the wait can be frustratingly long.

# DEALING WITH DISAPPOINTMENT

If fertility treatments fail, you're bound to be left feeling disappointed and inadequate. Even though you may be afraid of 'running out of time' and want to try again as soon as possible, you do need to recover physically and emotionally. Most reputable fertility experts recommend taking breaks between IVF attempts to allow your body time to heal. It would be a good idea to do a detox to rid your body of the aggressive chemicals and drugs you were given; the liver especially has been working hard to reduce toxins. After that nourish your body with the right food and exercise and try to find peace of mind through meditation or therapy. If you want to continue trying after a break, then it's important you remain positive. It can take more than one try for IVF to work, and the advantage the second or third time is that you're familiar with the procedures. This means you can focus on being receptive and calm rather than anticipating the next part of what is an invasive procedure. If you didn't have an accompanying course of complementary medicine to support treatment, you may want to try this next time. Also if you weren't happy with the way things were handled at the clinic, this is a good opportunity to try a different one. You may however decide, for whatever reasons, that you've had enough. This may come as a huge relief or it can take a long time to come to terms with.

## Moving On

Having a child is such a primitive drive and so rooted in society that the failure to do so can cause devastating psychological upset. Many women regard it as part of their blueprint for life to have children and it's still the norm in most cultures around the world. However, it's projected that a quarter of Britain's graduate women born in 1973 will remain childless.[7] Some women choose not to have children, but many never meet the right man, have numerous miscarriages or suffer failed IVF attempts. The loss of a dream child is very isolating because society has no processes or norms for dealing with the grief of childlessness like it has for other losses. There is also tremendous snobbery related to motherhood.

Believe me, if I hadn't written this book I'd have written the one about life without children. It can be just as fulfilling and maybe a bit more exciting, with the big advantage that you're more flexible. You have the luxury of spending time as you would like, you can go on holiday when and where you want, work as long or little as your needs require and you're financially much less compromised.

If you love children, then hopefully you'll have plenty of that energy in your life to bring you joy. All women are mothers to a certain degree, and many use their mothering qualities in caring for others. We each have our own personal journey and lessons in life which sometimes take to us to painful places. The best we can do is come out of suffering wiser, stronger and freer.

# CHAPTER 4

## When Something's Not Right

### PREGNANCY LOSS

Miscarriage is the shadow side of the bright and shiny subject of pregnancy. The news never finds us in pleasant places; caught out on a toilet discovering blood, or in an anonymous clinic watching a blurred image on a cold computer screen. No matter what anyone says – a baby you thought was coming has been lost. It already existed inside you; your future included this child – now, suddenly, these hopes and dreams are radically erased. It is a very lonely grief.

Motherhood begins the day you take responsibility for another being; this is often the moment you realize you're pregnant. It's your instinct to nourish and protect vulnerable life. To lose that fruit – however tiny it may have been – can bring up deep feelings of failure, guilt, helplessness and profound sadness. Aside from the physical and emotional trauma, pregnancy loss can make you question your sense of self. You are likely to feel inadequate and incomplete; maybe even ashamed of 'failing' in an essential female task. To *mis-carry* implies you've done something wrong, like you've let go of what you were meant to be holding.


## IT'S HAPPENING TO ME

### *Different Scenarios*

The medical term for bleeding and cramping in the first 20 weeks of pregnancy is *threatened abortion*. Bleeding in early pregnancy is actually very common, happening to 60–70 per cent of all women;[1] for half of those women it settles down and the pregnancy proceeds normally. Many doctors will tell you to lie down if you start bleeding. It's not proven this prevents miscarriage, but experts believe it can do no harm and keeps you calm. If bleeding does become heavier and the cervix is opening, there's little hope of saving the pregnancy and miscarriage is very likely; the medical term for this is *inevitable abortion*.

A *spontaneous abortion* is bleeding and cramping that leads to natural expulsion of the *products of conception*. If a scan shows all the tissue has been expelled, it's referred to as a *complete miscarriage*. If some of the pregnancy tissue remains in the womb, it's an *incomplete miscarriage*. The remaining tissue is usually expelled over time, but a later check-up is needed to make sure. If you get severe bleeding, cramps or a fever, it indicates infection, and medical or surgical treatment might be needed.

A *missed abortion* is where the foetus has died or failed to develop but your body has not physically expelled it yet. The pregnancy test may still show positive but you could have fewer pregnancy symptoms.

A *blighted ovum* is when the ultrasound shows an empty pregnancy sac; it may be because the fertilized egg did not divide and develop as it should have or the embryo stopped developing so early that it was absorbed into the surrounding tissue. You may still have some pregnancy symptoms.

You may feel these are all very harsh-sounding terms. You would be right. As I've mentioned, our society has no protocol for handling these types of loss.

### SIGNS OF A THREATENED PREGNANCY LOSS

- bleeding that becomes heavier
- severe cramping
- an open cervix
- pregnancy symptoms disappearing or weakening
- innate sense of sadness or rupture of 'link' with baby

## Miscarriage Management

The majority of miscarriages, around 95 per cent, occur in the first trimester. A most critical time in pregnancy is around week 10 to 12, when the embryo has formed most of its organs. This is also when the placenta takes over hormonal support from the *corpus luteum* (the follicle in the ovary from which the egg was released). If not before, this is the moment the body will register that the pregnancy isn't going ahead as it should and will begin the process of expulsion. It also explains why once you've passed the 12-week mark, your chances of miscarriage drop radically. This is why many people wait 3 months to go public with their baby news.

With today's technology, such as scans, we can find out early on if a foetus is viable and this has changed the way we experience pregnancy. It can be reassuring to know all is well at eight weeks. However, a bad scan result means you may end up with medical or surgical intervention, which can be harder on the body than a spontaneous abortion. Most doctors prefer to empty the womb to prevent the risk of infection which can occur if miscarriage is incomplete. And most women, naturally enough, want to get it over with if they find out they're carrying a dead foetus.

'For my first miscarriage I had to go into hospital for aspiration. I felt powerless and it brought up dark memories of an abortion I'd had when I was younger. It's like you go in full and still pregnant, they prise you open with their machines and you wake up very sore, numb and empty. When I miscarried spontaneously it was a process that started slowly with light spotting. Even though the uncertainty of whether I was miscarrying or not was hell, it did give me time to come to terms with the loss. On the fourth day of bleeding I got cramps, like period pains. It was very sad but my body recovered much faster than the time with intervention. I also felt more in control.'

REBECCA, MISCARRIAGES AT 37 AND 38, BABY AT 40

## *Late Miscarriage*

A late death of the foetus in the uterus after 20 weeks or at birth is referred to as a *stillbirth*. This is one of the hardest experiences for a mother to deal with. The main causes are infection, placental problems, malformations or complications with the umbilical cord. Any bleeding after the 28th week should always be investigated, as this could endanger the baby. *Neonatal death* is when a baby is born alive but dies within 28 days. The main causes of this are low birth weight and prematurity.

'I couldn't imagine ever getting through the pain of that loss and leading a normal life again. But slowly, little by little, the light began to shine once more. The wound has healed now, but it doesn't take much to reopen it.'

DINA, WHO HAD A STILLBIRTH WHEN SHE WAS 40

## UNDERSTANDING THE CAUSE

When miscarriage occurs, it's illogical but completely normal to blame yourself. You look for answers: why and what you could have done to prevent it. Around half of all miscarriages are due to chromosomal problems, and doctors say this increases with age (remember, computer programmes and charts work with chronological age rather than biological age). Nature's way of dealing with genetic malformations is to abort them. Other reasons for miscarriage could be:

- **Anatomical** problems with the cervix or uterus
- **Hormonal** factors due to polycystic ovarian syndrome, not producing enough progesterone to sustain the pregnancy or progesterone being blocked
- **Immunological** reasons – this is when the mother's body rejects the embryo as foreign tissue. Your blood can be screened for immune disorders and auto-antibodies, such as NK (Natural Killer) cells.
- **Environmental** factors such as smoke, drugs and drink – ones you can generally control.

Miscarriages can also be due to medical disorders such as heart disease, infections and everyone's favourite: stress.

*Recurrent miscarriage* is when you suffer three or more miscarriages back to back. Around 15 per cent of recurrent miscarriages are due to blood-clotting disorders, for which there are treatment possibilities.[2] In Western medicine they like to give mini-aspirin or heparin; the Chinese approach would be to prescribe herbs and acupuncture sessions. If women with this *Antiphospholipid syndrome* are treated, the live birth rate rises to 70 per cent.[3] With a new discovery called *Fertility Enzyme Therapy*, this figure rises to 79 per cent.

No matter how old you are, pregnancy loss is very common. Studies show that around 50 per cent of women suffer from one or more miscarriages, and at least 25 per cent of all pregnancies are lost. Early miscarriage often goes unnoticed or isn't reported, so there is little solid data on it, but experts suggest that around 45 to 75 per cent of all fertilized eggs are lost before implantation.[4] A miscarriage in its early stages is uncomplicated medically and usually experienced as a late, heavy period. It can become traumatic if you're trying hard for a baby and it keeps happening.

> *'Younger women miscarry, too, as most miscarriages are associated with chromosome abnormalities in the embryo which could be attributed to either the egg or the sperm. In my experience there's no evidence that older women are more at risk. From the patients I see, it's not necessarily the case. In your twenties maybe 90% of your eggs are good quality and ready for fertilization. Even if this declines with age, women will still produce good quality eggs but just less often than when they are younger, if they receive the help they need.'*
>
> DR XIAO-PING ZHAI, FERTILITY SPECIALIST

## Decreasing Your Risk of Miscarriage

There is a lack of treatment possibilities for miscarriage basically because there are few medical answers. Until you've miscarried three times, doctors won't investigate the causes, blaming it instead on 'random chromosomal error'. Even though this may be true for many cases, it isn't particularly reassuring or supportive in terms of knowing how to avoid further miscarriage. Chromosomal error basically means the DNA in the sperm or/and egg is damaged, causing the highly complex process of fertilization and cell division to fail. Scientists have just discovered that chromosomal errors in the eggs are probably due to a decrease in cohesion proteins which do the job of pairing off chromosomes correctly. Much of the DNA damage can be assigned to free radicals from our lifestyle and diet. Because our bodies have the ability to self-heal given the right conditions, there is in fact a lot you can do to improve your DNA and avoid miscarriage. There's a compelling study proving how pre-conception measures both restored fertility and eliminated miscarriage.

### ZERO MISCARRIAGES

One of the most comprehensive long-term studies ever conducted on fertility was carried out during a three-year period on 367 couples (654 individuals) by the University of Surrey and the UK charity Foresight. The test group ranged from 22 to 45 years, the average age being 35. Over a third of the couples had a history of infertility of up to ten years, 59 per cent had reproductive problems and 38 per cent had had between one and five miscarriages. Prior to the test period more than half of the couples smoked, 90 per cent of the men and 60 per cent of the women regularly drank alcohol. As part of the study the couples stopped smoking and consuming alcohol and followed a healthy diet; they bought organic food, ate more fruit and vegetables, cut down on caffeine, non-organic meat and dairy products. They also received individually tailored mineral and vitamin supplements. By the end of the three-year period, 89 per cent of the couples had given birth, including 81 per cent of those who had suffered infertility in the past. Most strikingly there were no miscarriages, premature births, perinatal deaths or birth defects. Based on average statistics for a test group this size there should have been 92 miscarriages, 11 birth defects and 5 stillbirths, but there were NONE.

## An Explanation

*'There is a good medical evidence base that the right diet, lifestyle and supplements can influence egg quality to improve fertility and avoid miscarriage. The follicle*

*has to mature in a healthy environment; this is a follicular fluid that bathes the egg in antioxidants. Down's syndrome is not inherited, it happens to the chromosomes at the time of fertilization. For healthy cell division there should be no blips on the DNA, as the cells divide and merge. Good nutrients are also important for the womb environment so the embryo ends up implanting. Toxins can impair all this.'*

DR MARILYN GLENVILLE

The cells surrounding the eggs also play an important role because they secrete the hormones required for proper functioning; a lack of the right hormonal environment can lead to more genetic irregularities.

## Reduce the Risks

- *Stop smoking* and avoid smoky environments – studies show that even exposure to second-hand smoke increases the risk of miscarriage.[5] Parental smoking is thought to produce the genetic breaks in sperm linked to miscarriage.
- *Stop drinking* – yep, afraid that even moderate drinking – as little as 3–5 units – has been shown to treble the risk of miscarriage in the first trimester.[6] Partners need to join your juice party; teetotal men have fewer damaged sperm.
- *Be caffeine-free* – reduce the amount of coffee you drink, ideally cut it out all together.[7]
- *No aspartame* – this nasty chemical is found in artificial sweeteners and diet drinks and has been linked to miscarriage.
- *Watch your weight* – being too under- or overweight will put you at risk of miscarriage.
- *Detox heavy metals* such as mercury, cadmium, lead and aluminium.

- *Neutralize stress* – get outside more, take breaks, start a social activity that doesn't involve alcohol, learn to meditate, have some holistic treatments, exercise regularly.
- *Increase blood flow and circulation* to your uterus through yoga, qi gong and massage.
- *Check nutrient deficiencies* – especially deficiencies in magnesium, selenium, beta-carotene, vitamins A, E, B$_6$, B$_{12}$ and omega 3, which are related to miscarriage.
- *Eat more organic fruit and veg* – a UK study of 7,000 women showed that those who ate fruit and vegetables regularly were 46 per cent less likely to miscarry. Women who lived near crops where pesticides were sprayed faced a 40 to 120 per cent increase in miscarriage risk.
- *Eat flaxseeds and sweet potatoes* – Sarah Dobbyn, author of *The Fertility Diet*, says this is her top nutritional counselling tip for women wanting to avoid miscarriage.
- *Maca* – a spoonful a day can help stimulate the pituitary gland, nourish the endocrine system and balance hormones.
- *Wild chasteberry* herb can help if you have low progesterone levels. It can be taken until the end of the first trimester to sustain the pregnancy.
- *Avoid dry-cleaners* – women working or living near dry-cleaners have higher miscarriage rates. Try to limit wearing chemically dry-cleaned clothes during early pregnancy or air them well before wearing.
- *Get psychological support* in early pregnancy, as this has been shown to increase the success rate by 86 per cent of women with unexplained miscarriage.
- *Have a medical check-up* to make sure you don't have any infections, parasites, genetic disorders or blood-clotting issues.
- *Practise positive thinking* – feeling strong, healthy and confident you will carry a pregnancy to term may increase your odds. There is still so much about miscarriage we don't understand.

RIGHT TIME BABY

Complementary medicine can also support your trust in your body.

- *Avoid pharmaceutical drugs and anti-depressants* – intake is linked to miscarriage.
- *Avoid canned foods and storing food and drink in plastic containers due to their bisphenol A (BPA) content* – women with recurrent miscarriage were shown to have higher levels of BPA in the body.
- *Avoid electromagnetic pollution* such as long periods spent at the computer without a break, using WiFi for extended periods, carrying your mobile phone on you or having long conversations on your mobile.
- *Avoid too many or long scans* – you will be encouraged to have additional scans if you've miscarried before to reassure you, but, ironically, scans have been linked to increased miscarriage rates.
- *Check your work environment* – flight attendants, anaesthetists and women working with chemical solvents, microelectronics, rubber, plastics or synthetics are all more susceptible to miscarriage.
- *Avoid street drugs* – this would seem obvious, but it also applies to partners. Cocaine use in males, for example, is linked to abnormal foetal development.

## GRIEF AND LOSS

*A Time to Cry*

Miscarriage can reopen old wounds or trigger memories of other losses we've suffered. These could be a previous miscarriage, abortion, death of a loved one or separation. The feelings of emptiness and isolation are very real.

Don't underestimate the importance of giving yourself the space to mourn and find the support you need. Girlfriends and female family members can be helpful, especially those who've

90

gone through a similar experience. You might want to perform your own closure ritual, such as burying the remains and planting a tree.

If you're a keen online chatter you could find solace in internet forums. Any type of bodywork, massage or healing will help you let go of pent-up sadness and anger.

## As a Couple

More often than not, women expect their partners to show a depth of understanding they're not able to communicate. You'll be on very different pages if you're feeling super-emotional and he's suppressing his feelings. Men generally tend to be more rational and detached in this kind of situation. Your partner may not want to be a burden to you, so by distancing himself it's his way of 'being strong'. Looking for distractions is another typical male way to deal with grief; in fact, many men don't grieve properly in the moment and end up carrying the scars for much longer than their partners, who immerse themselves in the pain. Of course it was *your* body carrying the baby and *your* body that's going through the hormonal changes, so it's bound to affect you more directly. For a man the difficulties include feeling like a bystander; he's powerless to prevent the events unfolding and protect his wife from physical and emotional pain. Rather than being disconnected try to understand and support each other. Both of you are feeling sad, angry and confused, so don't make it worse by asserting any blame or guilt. A pregnancy loss can bring you and your partner closer, if you're patient and kind to each other. Remember this is part of your collective story now as a couple.

## Simple Things for Him to Do to Make Her Feel Better

- Make sure she's warm and comfortable and fed. The sooner you pamper her, the sooner she'll pamper you back.

- Take her seriously even if you think she's acting barmy. Imagine your body being flooded with happy pregnancy chemicals and then suddenly the tap turns off and extreme sadness is pumped through your system.
- Let her cry as much as she wants without raising your eyebrows, giving her funny looks or turning the TV louder. Every so often give her a hug.
- Listen to her and don't offer comments like, 'It wasn't meant to be' or 'It would have been worse if you'd got to know the baby.' It might make sense to you but she wants her feelings validated, not hear comments a stranger could have made.
- If you have other children offer to take them out for a few hours, so she can have a bit of space.
- Use your pub allowance to buy her a massage voucher. It may feel painful at the time but you will go straight to heaven for this without passing through purgatory.

Understanding him: don't get cross if he does none of the above because he's 'too busy.'

## Sharing the News

When you've lost a baby you had your hopes on, telling other people may be the last thing you want to do. It stops you from *pretending* the diagnosis was all a mistake and that the foetus will wake up and start growing again. There's a great silence surrounding miscarriage, making it one of society's taboo subjects. People just don't know how to respond, apart from the usual embarrassed well-meaning comments like 'It was for the best.' There are no pregnancy loss cards like there are condolence cards for death and no specific mourning rituals. An invisible loved one who never 'lived' has died – it's such a hard concept for society to grasp.

Telling your boss and people at work why you need time off is particularly tricky. You may not want them to know you were trying to get pregnant, as this could affect your job or future career opportunities. This is really a case where lying is absolutely legitimate. You may have decided not to take a new job when you found out you were pregnant or made plans to take a sabbatical. Weeks and months of planning and reorganizing are altered again. It's a pain but that's life; constantly changing. There's nothing you can do but stay flexible and go with what you're bombarded with.

## HEALING AND HOPE

*Renew*

Mourning a pregnancy loss can take a while. A friend of mine found the physical discomfort the hardest aspect, whereas I found the disappointment took time to get over. Some women may find they feel better within weeks. Others need a few months. For some women it can take years – especially those who carried the baby to term or had a stillbirth. A miscarriage is something you never forget. It's branded into your personal and medical history; and it tragically drives home the fact of just how fragile human life is. But hopefully there will come a point when you're ready to move on.

After a miscarriage your body goes through a kind of purge. You can support the effect of this by doing a spiritual cleanse or healing. A friend of mine found it surprisingly difficult to recover from a miscarriage she had at 42 after finally meeting the right partner. A Family Constellations healing session was very helpful because it gave her some answers and freed up the tensions, expectations and fears she was feeling. Also, practices such as meditation and positive thinking really do influence our wellbeing, even if we engage just a few minutes a day.

If you decide you can't go through all that hope, excitement and disappointment again, then give yourself something to take your mind off things. Appreciating what you have helps you gain new perspective. You may still be childless but you have a wonderful circle of friends, or a fulfilling job you enjoy. By putting space between the event in the past and yourself in the now, things become easier. If you believe that everything is just the way it's meant to be, then hardship is easier to accept. People do resurface after tremendous loss; often as stronger and more compassionate beings.

> 'I was pregnant for about ten weeks, when the foetus died. But in that little time, I could already feel the distinct presence of another being with me. It wasn't my imagination, but a clear sense of connection, of holiness, that left me in awe. I guess I'll never give birth to a child, but I don't have the feeling that I've missed out. I experienced the most precious thing a woman can experience: to carry another life within her body, whether it lives to see the world or not.'
>
> CLAIR, 42, MISCARRIAGE AT 36

## Trying Again

Suffering from miscarriage may increase your desire to have a child. If you do decide to try again, the big question is when. A lot of this depends on how traumatic or complicated your loss was. If you were only pregnant for a short time, getting pregnant immediately should be all right. Most doctors say you can try as soon as you've had a healthy period, others suggest waiting two to three cycles. If your miscarriage was more difficult, it's better to give it a few months. According to Chinese and Ayurvedic medicine you need to recover properly first; this is because you lose a lot of blood during miscarriage and your body needs time to rebuild this supply and find balance. The Chinese also believe that having children too close together – even if you don't carry the pregnancy to term – reduces your life energy (they believe you need the Qi to anchor a new spirit). And don't forget the hormonal rollercoaster you go through every time. It can take 1 to 2 months for the pregnancy hormones to leave your bloodstream. Another good reason to wait is that it gives you a chance to do another pre-conception check and detox. This will help improve the quality and environment of your eggs and make sure you have all the nutrients you need for the next pregnancy. Don't forget your partner's sperm plays a big role, especially in older couples. Ideally wait 3 to 6 months to make sure egg and sperm are as strong as possible. At first this may seem like a long time if you're eager to get pregnant again but it passes very quickly once you're out of the immediate blue aftermath of miscarriage.

From my own experience and that of friends who've had miscarriages, a good six-month gap between pregnancies meant a successful outcome the next time round. Waiting also means you'll be more resilient because trying for a new pregnancy brings with it new possibilities of failure. If you had difficulties conceiving the last time, then it'll be harder to find the courage and willingness to start all over again. You're bound to feel burnt and apprehensive at least until your pregnancy goes beyond your last one. Try not to compare too much; feel positive about it, remember how the mind affects the body. Being pregnant again will support the healing process. Your chances of miscarriage don't go up if you've had a previous pregnancy loss. It's shown that 97 per cent of couples who suffer a miscarriage end up being parents, so the odds are definitely in your favour.[8]

# CHAPTER 5

## Pregnancy – The First Trimester

## PREGNANCY SIGNS

You generally do know before you know. Whether your pregnancy is planned or a surprise, the speculation can begin once you start getting these telltale signs.

### Temperature

For all those who've been charting their temperatures – this is where you can be cleverer than all the predictor kits. If your temperature stays high after ovulation, bingo, fertilization has taken place.

### Emotional

What might feel like PMT at first – a very dark, deep PMT – is your hormones getting the message there's a new body on board. Outbursts of tears and confused tantrums are your rite of passage into motherhood. Welcome!

## *Smells*

This is the first one that gets me every time. My nose morphs into a hypersensitive organ. Smells develop layers almost 3D-like with kaleidoscopic hues – no drugs involved, I promise, but increasing levels of oestrogen. Sometimes these new odours are so repulsive you feel the next thing in this list.

## *Sickness*

Whoever called it 'morning' sickness was having a laugh (or it was a male doctor who had obviously never been pregnant). Many of my friends and I suffered from all day and night nausea involving spontaneous dates with the toilet bowl. In most cases the sickness starts at about 6 weeks and abates around 3 months. But for that dreadful time you do wonder how anyone can possibly enjoy their pregnancy. There is no hard-and-fast rule as to who gets sick and why. If you're feeling abysmal, what might cheer you up is that it's actually a good sign because it means you're definitely pregnant.

## *Cravings and Aversions*

Everyone always talks about cravings (gherkins, chocolate cake, fish in brine – often in that order) but it's actually more common to be completely turned off certain foods. This can become a ridiculous cycle of nausea and hunger. If you could eat, you might not feel so sick but what on earth should you eat if everything turns you off?

## *Swollen Breasts*

A general lift upwards and outwards in the chest department may be visually appealing but rather painful. Your breasts have begun the journey from sexual playthings to what they were really made for: feeding a baby. Your partner may get frustrated by the new 'look but don't touch' rules, especially if you clobber him with the nearest sharp object every time he can't resist a little stroke. This will put him in good stead for the coming weeks when the above mentioned all-day sickness and exhaustion can put you off sex completely. However, some days your libido may skyrocket and that superfemininity you're exuding will make up for all the off days – at least that's what you should tell him.

## Glowing

Other people may notice this before you do – commenting on how radiant you are and how smooth your skin looks. Your cheeks take on a rosy, *just used the perfect blusher that was made to match my skin tone but no cosmetic company ever produces* tone. Wrinkles are smoothed out and you can actually appear about ten years younger. On the other hand your skin may go blotchy, spotty and dry – yep, life isn't fair; a cruel fact you should've realized by now.

## Contractions

A pulling sensation in your abdomen – a bit like a sharp instrument being dragged around your womb – is often mistaken as pre-menstrual pains. But in effect this is implantation taking place: the egg nestling into the lining of your uterus. It's not uncommon that implantation is followed by some light bleeding, also known as *spotting*. If you're trying to get pregnant, this pulling sensation is quite exciting and a sign that if you haven't already laid off the Mojitos, it might be high time.

## Busting to Go

This is only just the beginning of pregnancy-related incontinence. But there is good reason, because nature is perfect. The hormone relaxin, which allows your body to open for childbirth, is loosening the muscles, joints and organs, including the bladder. You may feel like a granny leaking all the way to the loo, but look on the bright side: countless toilet trips in the middle of the night will prepare you physically and psychologically for when the baby comes. One important thing to remember when you're out: use the toilet every time you spot one. Standing in a crowd with your knees pressed together might not be the look you want.

## Fatigue

Tiredness – sheer and utter exhaustion – is a sure telltale sign of a new pregnancy. It's a fatigue you may not have known previously and involves wanting and needing to fall asleep in the middle of meetings (hardly unprecedented!), sex (ditto?), conversations, films, train journeys and everyday chores that involve a certain degree of concentration. Increased levels of the hormone progesterone, and your body working hard dividing cells to create a new entity, are to blame for this chronic sleepiness. It's enough to make you demand a sabbatical. Usually this lethargy eases off after 3 months. But it's also a good excuse to put your feet up and read this book (until you nod off).

## Dizziness

If your head spins and your vision goes black from something simple like picking up a sock (even pregnancy won't stop your husband from being a slob), you're not necessarily hungover, but pregnant. I have a friend who mysteriously fainted and got herself a nasty black eye. It took her completely by surprise that her missed period was not early menopause (she was 43) but pregnancy.

## Heavy Legs

Increased blood pumping around your veins can cause painful swelling. It can be hereditary: my mother and grandmother suffered and reckoned it got worse with each pregnancy. Wearing compression tights may not be so sexy (and getting them on is like wrestling an elephant's trunk into a condom) but they can help hold back those varicose veins. A healthy diet and regular exercise will aid the blood flow, as will elevating your legs higher than your hips – there we go again, another excuse to put your feet up.

## Constipation, Bloating and Flatulence

All of these unpleasant ailments are very common because pregnancy hormones slow down your digestive system. A farting, belching female may not be so appealing, but then most of us have put up with farting, belching males all our lives. Isn't there some justice out there?

## Intuition

In modern society we have lost touch with this powerful tool, but when it comes to pregnancy women often do have a sixth sense. This *certain feeling* may also apply to others: I have often guessed when my girlfriends were pregnant, even before they knew it themselves (did I mention I'm probably psychic?).

## Missed Period

It may seem pretty obvious, but some women are so irregular they can't rely on their *friend* to cue them to pee over the predictor stick. Even if you're on the later side of late, you might not realize you're with child. Stay vigilant to the other signs and if in doubt run along to your local pharmacy to pick up a test. My friend Sigal did numerous tests for both her pregnancies, just to be sure. She still stores predictor packets in her bathroom, so if you live anywhere near Stoke Newington, pop along to her house, she's likely to have some spare.

If you only have some of the above signs, don't worry. Every woman is different and every pregnancy is unique.

## BABY

### *Month 1, Weeks 1 and 2*

Yes, I know you're not even pregnant yet. But this is officially where it all begins because they count the first day of your last period as the start of a 40-week pregnancy.[1] It will be the age of the uterus lining rather than the baby.

### *Month 1, Week 3*

This is usually, depending on ovulation, when conception occurs. After sperm meets egg, the fertilized cell keeps dividing to form a microscopic cluster of cells called a *blastocyst*. This ball of cells travels down your Fallopian tube to the uterus, sending out hormonal signals.

### *Month 1, Week 4*

The approximate week when the embryo, as it's now called, reaches the uterus and, attracted by proteins, snuggles itself or *implants* into the prepared uterine lining. Once in place the cells split again into two: the placenta and the embryo. The embryo – about the size of a poppy seed – has three layers. The inner layer, or *endoderm*, will develop into the baby's liver, lungs and digestive system. The middle layer (*mesoderm*) will become the heart, kidneys, muscles, bones and sex organs. The outer layer (*ectoderm*) will form the nervous system, hair, skin and eyes.

## Month 2, Week 5

The tadpole-like embryo is growing rapidly and is already the size of an orange pip. This week the circulatory system and heart are starting to form. Also the neural tube, which will eventually become the baby's brain and spinal cord, is developing.

## Month 2, Week 6

Measured from crown to rump (the tail or soon-to-be legs are still curled up) the embryo is now about 5–6 mm long and one month old. Eyes, ears, nose, jaw, cheeks and chin formation begin this week. The kidney, liver and lungs are also developing. The tiny heart is beating at 80 beats per minute.

## Month 2, Week 7

About the size of a blueberry, the embryo is now already 10,000 times bigger than at conception. Much of this growth is focused on the head area. New brain cells, the mouth and tongue are taking shape. Arm and leg buds are beginning to sprout and the kidneys are also preparing to start their function.

## Month 2, Week 8

We're now at large raspberry size, about 1.25 cm. The embryo's facial features continue to take more shape, as do its legs and back. The heart is beating at 150 bpm.

## Month 3, Week 9

About 2.5 cm in length – or the size of an olive – the future baby is now no longer called an embryo, but a foetus. Muscle formation begins this week.

## Month 3, Week 10

Nearly 4 cm long and similar to a prune in size, the foetus is developing knees, ankles and elbows. Bones, cartilage and buds of teeth are forming. The stomach has already started to produce digestive juices and the kidneys urine.

## Month 3, Week 11

Weighing about 8 g and measuring 4.5–6 cm, the body begins to straighten. Hair follicles, finger- and toenail beds are taking shape. In fact the little entity is beginning to look more human, with hands and feet, ears, a tongue, nipples and open nasal passages. If the foetus is a girl, ovaries start to develop.

## Month 3, Week 12

About the size of a plum, most of the foetus' systems are fully formed by now (and it's only 2 months old!). The digestive system begins contraction movements, the bone marrow is making white blood cells and the pituitary gland in the brain has started producing hormones. It will still take a while for the systems to mature, however.

## Month 4, Week 13

The foetus is between 6.5 and 7.8 cm long – the size of a peach – although its head is about half the length of crown to rump. Towards the end of the first trimester the vocal cords are forming. The placenta, which is the baby's life-support machine, is completely formed.

## Month 4, Week 14

Already fist-sized – around 8–9.3 cm and 25 g heavy (or light), the baby's features appear quite human. The eyes are now in the middle of the face, no longer on the side, and the ears are in their normal place, rather than the back of the head (!!) as before. The baby might even be growing some hair. The neck starts stretching and the head is more erect.

### Month 4, Week 15

Around 10 cm long and 50 g heavy – the size of an orange (we really are going through all the fruits here) – the baby's central nervous system starts controlling its reflexes and movements. It can move its arms and legs, curl its fingers and toes and even suck its thumb.

### Month 4, Week 16

Foetus sizes and weights differ, but they all develop along the same path from week to week. Your baby can now weigh between 80 and 142 g and measure from 10.8 to 13 cm. The muscles and movements are getting stronger, so that the baby is straightening out more. If you touch your belly, he or she will feel it. The baby is swallowing and excreting amniotic fluid and the kidneys have started working.

## ME

### Shiny, Happy Mummy

So you're pregnant. Wow! Even though it happens to women all the time, when it's happening to you, it's monumental. You are a mother fertile with new seed: femininity holding the secret of creation. Pregnant women are practically holy (and should be treated with particular TLC) because they're carrying precious new life. You literally have light within you. Your amazing body is growing another human being who'll be unique in every aspect (OK, I'll ease off. I think you get the picture!).

> *'Humans are an extraordinary mixture of earth and light; light, that is never as visibly radiant than during pregnancy. I would like to remind women that in these glowing months they are filled with life itself with all its strength and inexhaustible power.'*
> FREDERICK LEBOYER

For a woman who has sailed many oceans, you may suddenly find yourself in uncharted waters at the start of your biggest adventure yet. It's bound to affect you – and everything in your vicinity – in profound ways. For the next 9 months you'll perceive everything through your pregnancy glasses. And everyone else will perceive you shining with that certain, mysterious light – even on your bad days.

## HEALING LIGHT

Get some vitamin D from the sun by exposing yourself to natural light, especially bright morning light. A study showed that a couple of weeks of morning bright light therapy reduced depression in pregnant women.[2] Research also shows that sunlight plays an important role in the development of an unborn child's nervous and immune systems. Children of mothers who got little sunlight in the first 90 days of pregnancy were at an increased risk of getting multiple sclerosis later in life.[3] Researchers have also found that exposure to sunlight during late pregnancy helped children grow taller and have stronger bones.[4]

As an older pregnant woman you'll have heaps of expectations and fears. One minute you may be relieved your body's still capable, and the next you're worrying about absolutely everything from whether you should eat cheese to whether you can dye your hair.

The first few months of your pregnancy are the trickiest because they're the most uncertain and you're feeling ever so tired. Questions like: *Is the baby healthy? How do I cope with work and commitments? Will the baby's dad stay with me? Will childbirth hurt?* – all are completely sensible questions most pregnant women ask themselves, no matter what age they are. The first months aren't the most enjoyable. So hang on in there – it does get better.

## FIRST TRIMESTER CHEER-ME-UPS

- When you're sick, you've got the best excuse to eat exactly what you fancy (who cares if it's gherkins on a muffin?).
- You'll look pregnant soon and then everyone will treat you like royalty.
- You can get away with erratic behaviour: shoplifting, speeding and bouts of temporary insanity – well, at least you can try.
- Just take at look at your breasts: if that doesn't cheer you up enough, look forward to them getting even bigger and firmer.
- Enjoy the fact that your body is an intricately perfect creation and that everything you're feeling is happening for a reason in a miraculous process. See it as proof that women are, in fact, superior to men.

Even though you may feel so unbelievably weird, you don't actually *look* pregnant yet. So that is an added twist. You might start forgetting things, lose control of your emotions and find yourself with a kind of pregnancy dementia. My boyfriend would always notice this before I did (proving that barmy people never think they're barmy) and point it out in the least diplomatic ways (he's Spanish, so go figure!). It's particularly hard to make people understand why you're so moody and tired if you're keeping the pregnancy secret. If you've never lied before in your life, this may be the moment you start becoming an expert.

## LIST OF EXCUSES

- If eyebrows are raised when you refuse to drink, tell people you're avoiding alcohol as part of a special liver-cleanse which you do for a month so you can drink like a fish for the rest of the year.
- Get out of social commitments (and work) by saying you have an unusual strain of highly contagious flu requiring one week's incubation and at least an extra week to recover from the virus.
- When you're caught falling asleep at the keyboard at work, say you've found that dreaming on top of your project motivates you to excel in its execution.
- Refuse heavy lunches by saying you're on the latest diet from LA which involves bingeing on soda and breadsticks.
- Say you need to go home early because your relationship is going through a highly charged, passionate phase (then go home and straight to bed, whether he's lying in it or not).

## Telling Folk

Some women can't help spilling the good news to complete strangers on the bus. Others want to keep it from even close members of the family until it *just doesn't look like a weight problem any more*. Many people wait until the risky phase has passed (after 12 weeks). However, miscarriage is so traumatic anyway that you may want to let family and close friends know you're pregnant, so that they can be there to support you if something goes wrong.

## Possible Reactions

**Parents:** Relief – if it's your first baby – you've finally got there and they'll be promoted to grandparents after all. The announcement can produce slight weirdness because you're admitting that you engage in sexual activities and, despite what they may have thought, they now have to face the fact that you're no longer a virgin.

**Partners:** Mixed reactions from ear-to-ear grinning to worrying about the added responsibility, the end of his freedom and his pub money. Either way he'll have a glowing sense of pride that his semen is valid. NB If he's a modern man – or a control freak – he'll probably want to do the test with you and see that line for himself. Facing him with a *fait accompli* may cause considerable aggro.

**Girlfriends:** Whoops of joy. Women always love it when other women are gestating. Unless, of course, they're finding it hard to get pregnant themselves, then sharing the good news should be handled with discretion – and a box of tissues.

**Boss:** He or she will be officially supportive and unofficially pissed off, depending on how many other women from the team are on maternity leave.

**Work Colleagues:** Even if they smile and congratulate you, they're jealous they won't be taking time off, and worried they'll have to cover for you.

**Strangers:** Everyone loves baby news, but beware: some anonymous confidantes offer advice you don't need.

## Things to Consider Now

Should I tell people I'm pregnant? (see above)

Should I do the pre-natal tests? (read the next chapter)

When is the due date? (see below)

## DUE DATE CALCULATION

- According to Franz Naegele (1778–1851): first day of your last period minus 3 months plus 7 days and 12 months (doctors today still go by this fuddy old German's rule)
- If you know when you conceived, add 266 days (or 38 weeks)
- Remember: only 4 per cent of babies are born on their calculated due date, and 85 per cent are born within the two weeks before or after that date

# NURTURE

## *Love Your Food*

Enjoying nutritious food is the cornerstone of a healthy pregnancy. However, it's also a time when we can find it hard to control what we eat and become rather obsessive about meals (they became the highlights of my day; pity any mortal who got in my way). It's worth putting some thought and love into what you're ingesting because you are, after all, eating for two. Rather than eating more, this means eating better foods; quality not quantity counts. Sometimes during pregnancy our bodies crave certain foods and often these do contain things our body lacks (how does this work with doughnuts?). If you're new to healthy eating, don't give yourself too much of a hard time but do try to wean yourself from junk to nutrient-dense food. Think of it as a unique, and maybe once-in-a-lifetime, opportunity to really look after yourself.

## JUNK-FOOD ADDICT

If you're used to a diet of fast food then it will be quite a challenge to switch to more natural-tasting food. Processed foods contain a lot of salt (the wrong kind), sugar, fat and flavour enhancers, which make them addictive. They also numb your palate to other foods. But once you switch to wholefoods and notice how you have more energy and fewer digestive problems, your cravings for junk food should disappear.

## Some General Pointers

Eating well is important during pregnancy because your body needs more protein, vitamins and minerals such as calcium, iron, magnesium, folic acid, zinc and essential fatty acids (EFAs). The Standard UK Diet (SUKD) is low in EFAs, vitamins, minerals, antioxidants and water. There are many pregnancy supplements out there, but your digestive system needs to be working well to absorb these multivitamins. Many women like to take them as a back-up – but don't rely on them and remember: it's a supplement, not a 'substitute'. Getting nutrients directly from food is still the best way.

If you follow the advice on nutrition in Chapter 2 then the same basically applies. Eat fewer processed, refined foods and more wholefoods such as wholegrains, vegetables and fruit – organic if you can. If you eat meat then try to buy only organic meat for the pregnancy period to avoid the hormones, antibiotics, growth enhancers and GMOs (genetically modified organisms). If you're vegetarian or vegan make sure you up your intake of vitamin $B_{12}$, zinc, calcium and vitamin D (more about this in Chapter 8).

## Sick as a Retching Dog

During the first trimester it's often hard to eat well, especially if you're feeling sick. This is no cause for alarm because the growing embryo/foetus will take all the nutrients it needs from your stock (just make sure you build up your stock again when you're well). It is important you stay well hydrated, especially if you're actually vomiting. A key to good hydration is using real salt. Himalayan salt or unprocessed sea salt is not stripped of the vital minerals our bodies need and will help the body to absorb water.

Around three-quarters of all gestating women suffer from pregnancy sickness. There are various theories as to why this occurs, including raised hormone levels, fatigue and emotional stress. In some primitive societies morning sickness is unknown, which leads nutritionists to think that sickness is a reaction to the toxicity in our bodies and thus has a detoxing function.

## Sickness Cures

- Eat small meals at regular intervals – it is better to eat six small meals, than three big ones.
- Start the day slowly and eat something before you get up – breakfast in bed, yeah!

### The Following Foods Can Help

- Ginger – relaxes the stomach; put a slice under your tongue, eat it raw, candied, as a biscuit, drink it as tea, whatever you can get your hands on
- $B_6$ – found in nuts, bananas, avocados and wholegrains. If taken as a supplement, choose a pregnancy one containing no more than 10 mg
- Iron-rich food – leafy greens, eggs and sardines
- Dried apricots
- Pumpkin seeds
- Dry crackers
- Fresh mint as tea or on food (try sniffing it also).

### Try

- Acupressure bands – used by seasick sailors (an oxymoron if ever there was one!), these miracle armbands put gentle pressure on the points to relieve nausea

- Acupuncture sessions – your therapist will know which points to needle; ask to be shown how someone else can massage the points for you
- Aromatherapy oils – ginger, chamomile and lavender – as a room spray
- Wearing compression tights – they allegedly stabilize your blood pressure
- Getting some fresh air
- The homeopathic remedy *Nux vomica*.

## STRETCH

### *Couch Potato*

Pregnancy is the time to give up control a little. It's the best excuse to take it easy physically. Gentle forms of exercise like yoga, tai chi, qi gong, swimming, walking and dancing are perfect. Rigorous, strenuous exercise with jerky, forceful movements is not ideal when you're pregnant. Do what you personally feel is right for you. If you've been a runner all your life, you might not want to stop now. Just remember, don't push yourself too much and back off training for the Olympics, especially in the first months when your body needs to be nourished rather than exerted.

### *Yogi Mummy I*

Your hormones are making your body squishier and more flexible – perfect for pre-natal yoga. If you're a yoga virgin, this is a great time to start, and many women do discover yoga after they get pregnant. Some instructors say it's the best time in your life to do yoga because you're particularly in tune with its teachings and philosophy. If you're already a yogi, this is a great chance to deepen your practice.

Yoga connects you to your body and allows you to be really present; it encourages relaxation, focus and attention to breathing. This increases the amount of oxygen you and your baby are getting and improves circulation. Yoga is all about bringing yourself into awareness and balance. It is not a competition and you can't lose or win at it (although some people do try!).

In the first trimester yoga should be gentle and nurturing, rather than fast, strenuous and hot (so ease off the Bikram, hotties!). If you have a regular self-practice, try to take it a little slower, avoid deep twists, 'eagle' and any positions that compress your belly. Also avoid Kapalbhati breath and any cleansing or detoxing exercises. Focus more on nurturing postures and gentle Ujjayi breath. Some ante-natal yoga teachers won't take pupils until they've passed the 12-week mark, so you might be on your own if you're new to practising. There are some excellent pregnancy yoga books with photos and diagrams by Uma Dinsmore-Tuli, Françoise Barbira Freedman and Janet Balaskas. It's partly thanks to these teachers that ante-natal yoga has been given structure and made so accessible and effective.

*'When I started giving pregnancy yoga classes in the eighties, they said yoga was harmful.'*

FRANÇOISE BARBIRA FREEDMAN

*'I'm delighted that ante-natal yoga is so popular now. It is an ancient practice coming back to life, that pregnant women have known before, in matriarchal times. Yoga is deeply empowering in pregnancy as it connects us to the earth, deepens awareness of breathing, releases tension and helps you to connect with your unborn baby. There is no better way to prepare for the inner focus you will need for birth and the joy of becoming a mother.'*

JANET BALASKAS

## RELAX

### Meditating Mum

When you're pregnant, being able to relax can make all the difference. Most of us have to continue with our hectic lives as before, which is why taking time out to meditate can massively improve the quality of your pregnancy. It can help you manage the turbulent emotional aspect of gestation because you learn how to let go; this means you stop identifying with bad events. The goal is to achieve effortless concentration or relaxed awareness. You'll also find that meditation gives your brain a greater capacity to focus and deal with challenges even in a very stressful, hectic environment.

You can meditate anywhere, from a crowded train to an office desk; without anyone else noticing, you can just drift off to nirvana. To meditate in a focused way, however, it's best to take yourself to a quiet, comfortable spot for about 20 minutes; this can be soon after you get up in the morning, any time during your day or shortly before going to bed. The pregnancy hormone, progesterone, has a calming and soothing effect, so if you've never meditated before, it might actually be easier now.

---

#### POSITIVE EFFECTS OF MEDITATION FOR THE BABY

All the biological and psychological benefits of meditation are transmitted through your bloodstream to the womb and by so-called *sympathetic resonance*, a kind of telepathic and energetic communication you have with the baby. When you meditate adrenalin and cortisol levels are lowered, endorphins are released and melatonin and DHEA hormones are strengthened. This is a major boost for both the baby's and your own immune system. Regular meditating reduces blood pressure and lowers the risk of pre-eclampsia.[5] Meditation during pregnancy has been shown to reduce the need for pain-relief during birth – such as epidurals – by 85 per cent, and halve the number of caesarean sections.[6]

---

## A Little History and Science

Meditation goes back thousands of years to the ancient Vedic times in India. In fact yoga *asana* (the 'exercises') were developed as a way of preparing the body to sit for a long time in uncomfortable postures. Pregnancy yoga classes spend longer on meditation or yoga *nidra* (in comfortable, preferably lying-down postures) so you may learn what you need there.

The mind constantly looks for distractions – it wanders. You have thoughts about what you will do later, or what happened earlier that day, for example. Westerners find it particularly difficult to stop the constant chatter of the so-called *monkey mind*. During meditation you're basically 'stilling the restless mind'. You can distract it by giving it something to focus on such as a flame, your breath, sound or a mantra. Scientists have proven that meditation quite literally slows down the brainwaves. It also improves the structure of the brain: those who meditate regularly are shown to have more interconnected pathways.

### THE SCIENCE OF MEDITATION

**Beta waves** (13–38 Hz) occur when you're thinking and problem-solving. Stress and insomnia are at the high end (around 38 Hz) and concentration the low end (around 13 Hz).

**Alpha waves** (8–13 Hz) occur when you're relaxed and calm. Around 8 Hz you're almost asleep.

**Theta waves** (4–7 Hz) occur when you're deeply relaxed, dreaming and sleeping.

Pure meditation is when you're on the edge of alpha and theta: surfing the wave, so to speak. But even if you can only reach alpha you're still meditating and slowing down the brainwaves related to stress. The problem is when you get stuck in beta and the beta brainwaves dominate your life (know that 'mad' feeling?)

## GLOW

### Forget the Frump

Once upon a time a woman with child would do the utmost to cover her swollen belly. She'd wear shapeless, unflattering dresses, morphing into Pizza the Hut the more her mountain grew. Sexy and pregnant were a dichotomy. Think Princess Diana in her tent-like pinafores with those hideous frilly collars. No wonder she got depressed post-partum.

But gestating women this side of Neneh Cherry can breathe a deep, belly-rippling sigh of relief. That funky chick who rapped on stage with midriff pants, short tank top and the cutest pregnant tummy on display, changed the face of maternity wear forever. Well, not just her: there was also Demi Moore (doing her thing for the swollen belly rather than actual clothes), Gwen Stefani (in those pretty ethnic gowns, gathered flatteringly under the bust) and of course Angelina Jolie (who managed to look elegant even with a twin bump). The pregnant shape is now celebrated; it has become a stylish woman's most coveted accessory. Today you can buy everything from hip maternity jeans to cute breastfeeding bras in your favourite high-street store as well as from high-end designer boutiques.

### Madonna and Co.

Celebrities are a hard act to follow but you can look like a million dollars without necessarily having them (and the umpteen stylists that come with them). Take a tip from überfrau Claudia Schiffer who simply bought trendy clothes a few sizes bigger; this way she could stay faithful to her favourite designers throughout her last pregnancy at sexy 39 (interestingly she also did a Demi and bared her naked bump for German *Vogue*). Other LATER mums we may call style icons for maternity frocks are Heidi Klum, Halle

Berry, Jennifer (JLo) Lopez, Salma Hayek, Liz Hurley, Madonna, Nicole Kidman (gosh it just doesn't stop) and the sultry Italian actress Monica Bellucci, who has now had her second later baby at 45.

In the beginning you can probably still wear most of your normal clothes. Avoid the flared maternity look if you're keeping the pregnancy secret, because it's like an American tourist on the Tube – i.e. not very subtle. If you find you have to leave the top button of your trousers open (even before the rather filling meal) you might want to get some pregnancy jeans or trousers, with stretchy waistband. These are a worthwhile investment because they grow with you. T-shirts, shirts and jumpers will tighten suggestively over ample bosoms. This could be an image you quite like (your partner probably will) but if you feel like splashing out on something new, just buy a bigger size or a baby doll. If you're feeling shapeless, wear a long scarf to cover your middle bit. Tunics and kaftans can also camouflage a disappearing waistline with flair. Anything that is three-quarter length or longer will work. Anything that accentuates your bust will distract attention away from other bulges. If in doubt wear black, which can look very chic – although be warned, also terribly dull, depending on your hormonal state.

## LOVE

### Pregnant Papa

Relationships change when you're pregnant. You may feel closer to your mother, more affectionate with your cat, very intimate with your fridge – and there's a chance that you become more loved up about your partner, that heroic specimen of a man who got you in this wonderful predicament. If he's gentle and understanding about your sudden Brando-esque attacks of anger or Big Brother-style emotional outbursts, then he's already scoring lots of Brownie points, putting him in very good stead for perfect fatherhood and other shiny medals. However, most mortal men will be confused and unable to keep up with the rapidly advancing pace of pregnancy and your metamorphosis into a giant aubergine. This is a journey for both of you. It will bring you closer than you've ever been and it is likely to provoke the kind of arguments you previously only experienced in films (those where a spouse gets murdered). Reminding him he shouldn't upset a pregnant woman will only make matters worse.

## Sexy Mama

Pregnant sex is different to regular sex. It's either/or: you either don't care much for it (in a 'really couldn't give a damn' way) or you desperately crave it with such lust you scare yourself – and the neighbours. There's no middle way. Some women go one way, some the other, but most go to both extremes – depending on momentary mood and hormones. My friend Lydia felt like the holy virgin (literally) during her first pregnancy. Much to the dismay of her partner she insisted on keeping her immaculacy intact until well after the birth. But during her second pregnancy she became the gestating whore; sex was so hot she couldn't get enough of it. (Yep, you guessed it – she did have a Catholic upbringing.)

The first trimester is likely to be more erratic than erotic. First of all there's the fatigue. Your main desire is for sleep, not sex; you crave endless slumbering days and nights of it. Intercourse with a comatose woman on a sofa can lead to a prison sentence, so that will put most horny spouses off. Then there is nausea to contend with. When you're trying to hold down food, the last thing you want is more meat (*pardonnez-moi!*) forced into another crevice of your body. For me personally it was smells that had me running. I suddenly developed this aversion to male body odour, including my freshly showered lover's. I also have friends who went off sex because it seemed pointless. The baby's already in there, DUH, oven's full.

## MYTH: HAVING SEX CAN LEAD TO MISCARRIAGE

Unless you have a history of miscarriages or are bleeding, there's no reason to refrain from penetrative sex in the first trimester.

If you can actually find a milli-second in the day when you're not feeling tired, sick or too philosophical about the meaning of life, then sex may be fabulous. The fact that you're pregnant can be a huge turn-on. You may feel earthy and sensual, fulfilling an innate fecundity. Big daddy may feel more virile in a swaggering sort of way (and massively relieved he's not firing blanks). Many men are said to fantasize guiltily about other women when their wives are pregnant. My partner said he started seeing women as potential females to impregnate rather than just have sex with. Charming! Rather than take this personally (unless he does go and 'spread his seed') see this as a reminder that man (and sometimes woman) is in fact an animal with very basic instincts.

## THE FIRST TRIMESTER FOR HIM

- It takes him 3 months to get over the shock and used to the idea that he's definitely no longer a single man – even if he's been married 5 years.
- He's also *feeling* pregnant. Higher levels of prolactin and oestrogen – hormones that stimulate motherly bonding behaviour – are found in the saliva of partners of pregnant women. But the big difference is he won't get any extra attention or have good excuses like feeling tired or sick.
- He can't understand why you burst into tears so easily and forget everything. But he's secretly worried you were abducted by aliens and replaced with a faulty clone.

## WORK

### Pulling Sickies

For most of us, getting pregnant doesn't change our everyday commitments, especially the money-making ones. It would be such a perfect world if the blue line on your pregnancy test meant immediate release from all duties and a free ticket to Hawaii. There's clearly no justice in getting on an overcrowded bus with morning sickness and dragging yourself to an airless office when you really need to go back to bed (and read baby books like this one all day). Come on, drama queen! Grit your teeth, hard shoulder to the wheel, the economy needs you! If you really are too sick or tired to cope, and the measures mentioned below don't help, try to get a doctor's note until you feel stronger. However, there are a number of pregnancy complications (diabetes, high blood pressure, history of miscarriage and expecting multiples) that entitle you to sick leave.

You may be outraged that I would even suggest you missing a day's work. Hopefully you love your job so much and have such important responsibilities (you're prime minister, are you?) that your main concern is being able to combine work with pregnancy. Multi-skilling was invented by mothers, so as a gestating female you have the best prerequisite. But do pace yourself, especially if you have a tendency to overdo it or push your limits. Remember that your health and the baby's come first, so try to avoid stress.

#### HOW TO MANAGE WORK DURING PREGNANCY

*Get plenty of rest.* Generally you need at least 8 hours' sleep. If this means early nights, do it! Midday naps are also very regenerative; if it's warm enough, take lunch in the park and have a snooze; in colder or wet weather book a massage or treatment so you can lie down and sneak in a kip. If your workplace has a sofa somewhere private, lie down.

*Eat well.* Try to eat a healthy breakfast with wholegrain carbs, prepare a juice for mid-morning, eat lunch plus a mid-morning and mid-afternoon snack, always carry water and keep nutritious nibbles (fruit, vegetable sticks, nuts, crackers with tahini and cereal bars) in your desk and bag.

*Take regular breaks.* If you work long hours at a computer, take short office strolls every 30–40 minutes; you can go to the loo, which you probably need to do anyway.

*Put your feet up.* Try to find a stool, box or bin to elevate your legs and feet; bring cushions to sit on and support your back. If you have to stand for long periods, wear those sexy support tights, keep one bent leg on a stool and alternate legs to take pressure off your back. Sit down when you can (bring a fold-up stool if necessary).

*Get some fresh air.* Definitely in your lunch break, and mid-morning and mid-afternoon would be ideal as well. Take deep breaths to fill your lungs with oxygen (inner-city ladies: choose to do this near plants, not the bus exhaust fumes).

*Move and stretch regularly.* Keep the blood moving; stretch your arms above your head; point your toes; rotate wrists and ankles; roll your head in a circle in both directions. Those in 'snigger-free' environments can do some simple yoga postures like standing bent forward against your desk to stretch the back, or the posture Downward Dog.

*Reduce on-the-job stress.* Close your eyes and imagine yourself being in a relaxing place; put on some headphones and listen to music; daydream and enjoy your day.

*Dress comfortably.* Wear loose rather than restrictive clothing, flat shoes and layers so you can adapt as your body temperature fluctuates (sweat, freeze, freeze, sweat).

*Keep well hydrated.* Drink plenty of water and herbal teas. Cut out coffee, black tea and fizzy drinks.

*Reduce duties at home.* There's nothing worse than coming home to more work. Try being less of a perfectionist. If you have a partner, get him to help with housework and cooking. If you can afford it, get a cleaner. If you have other children and a lazy husband, run off to Siberia.

The main disadvantage of keeping your pregnancy secret at work is that you'll be expected to function as normal. Depending on how you're feeling and what type of work you do, you might want to 'come out' to your employer sooner rather than later. Your decision will also depend on whether reviews, buyouts or threatened redundancies are coming up. If you work for a family-friendly company you probably can't wait to tell them that you're ready for the bunch of flowers and the flexi-hours. There's more about 'going public' at work in Chapter 7.

### LEGAL LIES

If you're applying for a job or being interviewed for a new position you don't have to disclose you're pregnant. In fact you can deny it, even if they ask you. This is part of the law which states that pregnant women cannot be discriminated against. You also can't be fired because you're pregnant.

## WORRY LESS

If you're a later mother there's always someone ready to share a horror story with you. It should be officially registered as a crime to worry a pregnant woman. Pregnancy is hopefully a time of great health, but due to added strain on the body there are some common pregnancy ailments that might put the fear in you. You can't take the usual drugs because pharmaceuticals have side effects and could harm the baby – and that thought puts the fear in you even more.

If you're new to complementary or holistic medicine, then pregnancy can be a great catalyst. The beauty of holistic therapies is that they're individually tailored and have no negative side effects, so they are perfectly safe for you and your nestling. Being treated holistically will give you a greater understanding on how your body works – it's bound to be an enlightening and empowering experience. If you'd like to get a complete assessment try to find a therapist trained in various areas, such as a good naturopath. Many therapies have the pleasant 'side effect' of making you feel very relaxed, and this is bound to be good for baby-in-womb.

## Common Early Pregnancy Concerns

### Dizziness
This is due to your blood supply having to meet the new expanding needs of your circulatory system. It is important to keep blood sugar levels stable by eating small, regular, high-protein meals. You can also try drinking lemon balm tea or inhaling lavender essential oil. Hot/cold showering, dry brush rubbing and homeopathic remedies are also known to help.

### Constipation
As the muscles around your bowel begin to relax (and later there is pressure from your expanding uterus) constipation becomes quite a common problem in pregnancy. You can prevent it by exercising regularly and eating a high-fibre diet; ideally lots of uncooked fruit and vegetables, prunes, kiwis, linseeds, beetroot, cabbage and wholegrains. You also need to make sure you're drinking plenty of water. Avoid refined foods such as white bread and white rice as these will clog you up more. If you're taking an artificial iron supplement this could also be causing the problem; switch to a natural one such as *floradix* and eat more iron-rich foods. Try massaging your abdomen in a clockwise direction. Acupuncture

can help restore the natural action of the colon. An Ayurvedic remedy is drinking a cup of hot milk with ghee before bed. (See also the section on food combining in Chapter 8.)

## Headaches

Hormonal changes, tension, tiredness, dehydration, hunger and bad posture may all lead to headaches. Resting in a darkened room, going for a walk in the fresh air and doing something meditative can help. Often you might just want to go to bed because a headache can be a sign that you need more rest. Some headaches are due to a drop in blood sugar levels so remember to eat regular meals. Cold and hot compresses on the area that's painful are good remedies, as well as taking hot and cold showers. Try massaging lavender or peppermint oil onto your temples. Acupuncture, acupressure, massage and biofeedback are also recommended.

## Bleeding

Unbelievably scary when it happens because when we see blood we immediately think we could be losing the baby. In some cases it does mean miscarriage, but bleeding or spotting needn't necessarily be cause for alarm. It happens to many women and has various causes. If it happens in the first months and is not related to implantation, it could be that your cervix has been irritated due to a vaginal exam or intercourse. It can also mean you have a vaginal infection. Or it could be simply bleeding around the time of your usual period as your hormones are still unsettled. A check-up with a scan can be reassuring but it won't make the blood stop. If you ask the doctor they will often prescribe bed rest or tell you to take it easier. My friend Nathalie had quite heavy bleeding around her tenth week. The doctor confirmed everything was fine with her pregnancy and an appointment with a kinesiologist put it down to emotional stress due to worrying about the future, her relationship and how a second baby would change everything. In the end it was fine and she had a healthy baby girl.

A further (scientific) explanation for bleeding is that between weeks 10 and 12 the placenta takes over hormonal support from the corpus luteum in the ovary. The bleeding is not coming from the foetus but from the still-unoccupied uterine lining. This in no way presents a danger to the developing life.

If the bleeding is more serious, however, it needs checking urgently as it could indicate a miscarriage; there is more about this in Chapter 4.

# CHAPTER 6

## Tests and Decisions

### TO TEST OR NOT TO TEST

*Ante-natal (s)Care*

There was no free healthcare for women in the UK until the 1940s, but now we've gone to the other extreme. It's like you're signing up for the 25th infantry division. They want to prod, pin and puncture you, inspect your blood and analyse your urine. The 'industrialization of obstetrics' is what Dr Michel Odent – a world authority on childbirth and health research – calls it.[1] As soon as you get pregnant you're drawn into this unshakeable, invasive monster of a system that's focused on potential problems.

The belief that more ante-natal tests mean a better outcome for mother and baby is not based on scientific data. Studies have found that starting pre-natal care late or having a reduced visit schedule had no adverse effects.[2] This is why various experts today call for routine medicalized pre-natal care to be reconsidered. Depending on your healthcare provider, pre-natal appointments can actually cause more anxiety, because with each test there is another opportunity to worry about the results. Many doctors still see you at risk of complications if you're having a first baby over 35, despite the fact that there is little medical proof to support this pessimism. Various studies show that this 'high-risk' label causes fear-induced stress and increased emotionality in patients. The attitude of practitioners was found to contribute to, rather than ameliorate, complications.[3] There is also the danger that an over-medicalized pregnancy will end up in an over-medicalized birth.

In many cultures and societies, upsetting a pregnant woman is frowned upon. Both in Chinese and Indian traditions the community is to protect a pregnant woman so that she feels relaxed and happy. They believe that mothers and babies are directly linked, and everything that affects the mother will affect her unborn child. In the West we have to prove everything first before we believe it. Thanks to increasing data now available in the area of foetal origins we are learning that health is shaped to a great extent in the womb and that the emotional states of a pregnant woman influence foetal development. Stress, for example, leads to higher levels of cortisol, and this can inhibit foetal growth and brain development.[4]

Instead of money spent on expensive medical tests and scans, women would be better off with a personally tailored nutrition plan and having paid yoga classes, group swimming sessions, massages and other treatments that make them feel good and positive about this remarkable and unique time in their lives. Rather than being worried by unnecessary medical procedures, wouldn't it be more effective to see a supportive midwife who is trained in the more spiritual aspects of her wonderful profession? I'm sure the babies would prefer this to an ultrasound.

'I felt very strongly that I was the guardian of my womb and that it was my job to protect my child from all those needles and pins. Rather than scans I regularly went to a hypnotherapist who I knew could take me to a deeper level. I feel most of my mothering work was done while my daughter was in the womb. It was my responsibility to give her an emotional foundation of security and safety, not fear.'

**SHILPA, HEALTHY BABY AT 39**

## Unnecessary Routine Tests

Most women have a blood test to detect anaemia, but this gives a false diagnosis because it isn't taking into account the increased blood volume of pregnancy.[5] Pharmaceutical iron supplements are then prescribed which often produce constipation, diarrhoea and heartburn and inhibit zinc absorption.[6] Get iron in a balanced way through food or, if there really is reason to believe your iron levels are too low, take a plant-based iron supplement such as *floradix*. Acupuncture, acupressure, massage and reflexology can also improve blood flow and iron absorption.

Most women have increased blood pressure in late pregnancy and are wrongly told they are at risk of pre-eclampsia. You only have pre-eclampsia if there is more than 300 mg of protein in the urine every 24 hours. Increased blood pressure without protein in the urine is actually linked to good birth outcomes.[7]

If you belong to the tiny minority of women – around 3 per cent – who test positive for gestational diabetes, you will merely be given the standard advice any pregnant woman should get on exercising regularly and avoiding too much refined sugar, refined carbohydrates and soft drinks.[8]

## Striving for Perfection

Pre-natal diagnosis is another conflictual story. On one hand it's seen as a kind of safety net, or medical thumbs-up, to anyone who might be concerned about the health of their child. This can be particularly reassuring if you're over 35 because that's when they start waving the statistics at you. On the other hand the tests create their own risks, problems and uncertainties which taint the experience of pregnancy.

The invasive pre-natal tests with more definite results can't be done until about week 14. If you decide to have an amniocentesis, for example, it means you're in limbo for nearly half your pregnancy. It's hard to embrace a pregnancy that hasn't been deemed 'viable' yet.

No one *chooses* to have a baby with birth defects, so quite naturally every mother-to-be gets anxious when she's told her age could be a problem. In our paranoid, high-tech society, the risks are often overemphasized. There is a general bias towards doing more testing, even though 96–97 per cent of children are born perfectly healthy. The doctors aren't to blame for the scaremongering, because they're also afraid. They don't want to be accused – in extreme cases with legal action – of failing to warn future parents of any potential birth defects. This culture of fear is not conducive to anyone sleeping more soundly. And it certainly isn't doing much to facilitate the bonding process between mother and baby in utero.

> *'These examinations are never in the interest of the child. It is merely for selection purposes to see if it looks healthy. I don't know how this constant checking and analysing affects an unborn child.'*
>
> CORINNA, INDEPENDENT MIDWIFE WHO RUNS
> HER OWN BIRTHING CENTRE

Pre-natal diagnosis has its roots in the eugenics movement; so-called 'attempts to improve the race and its genetic make-up'. It asks for tricky judgements about whether a life is worth living. By introducing the dilemma of abortion early into the experience of motherhood it brings negative emotions into what should be a joyful time.

None of the tests are compulsory by law and you must give informed consent for the diagnostic ones.

> ### THINK ABOUT IT
>
> A 40-year-old is generally told she has a 1 in 100 chance of having a baby with trisomy (see page 140 for more about trisomy). If someone told her she had a 99 in 100 chance of winning the lottery, you bet she'd go and buy a ticket.
>
> A woman's body miscarries 95 per cent of chromosomally flawed pregnancies; an embryo with trisomy has less than 5 per cent chance of surviving until birth.[9]

Out of all the 'high-risk' women undergoing pre-natal diagnosis – and being over 35 is classified high-risk when it comes to birth defects – more than 95 per cent will get a reassuring result that the unborn baby doesn't have any of the disorders tested for.[10]

## ULTRASOUND

### Baby Pics

Otherwise known as a sonogram, a scan involves the transmission of high-frequency sound waves. A pattern of echoes from different surfaces such as fluid, soft tissue and bones from inside your womb are translated into images on a screen. Don't expect high-res quality footage of your little precious – it's more like a fuzzy, hard to distinguish picture. For most of us in our visually literate society, this is when pregnancy becomes real. It's the first snapshot you'll see of your baby and can be a hand-holding moment with your partner (or healthcare provider, if you're alone). It can help the bonding process, especially for fathers. Ask for a print-out because it will get plenty of mileage with family and friends, and nicely decorate the fridge door.

Ultrasound is performed by running a wand or transducer over your jelled-up belly. Sometimes, for a more exact reading, the dildo-like contraption is placed into your vagina and moved around a bit (this is your chance, just in case you forgot, to remember how the baby got there). The wand gets a hygienic, fresh condom rolled over it and a squirt of slippery gel. This little 'dressing the wand' ritual can provide mild entertainment if attempted by fumbling hands.

Ultrasound is sometimes performed early in pregnancy to confirm its viability. A gestational sac can be seen as soon as four weeks since your last period, and the foetal heartbeat can be picked up by some machines at 6 weeks. Scans are routinely used at around 12 weeks to screen for birth defects.

Sometimes a *Detailed Anomaly Scan* is performed after 22 weeks. This screening can detect structural malformations but cannot exclude chromosome abnormalities. Ultrasound is also used to calculate the due date of the baby by measuring it, although some experts believe this contributes to the increasing birth induction rates. Your doctor will be able to inspect foetal organs, the baby's position for birth and how the placenta is placed. A good guesser will be able to inform you whether you should buy pink or blue socks.

Going for an ultrasound can be more nerve-wracking than opening an envelope with exam results because it will tell you if something is wrong. If, for example the embryo has stopped developing, you will be told the devastating news on the spot.

## How Safe Is Ultrasound?

Most healthcare providers will assure you that ultrasound is perfectly safe. Although it has become a routine procedure over the last 20 years, latest findings indicate that scans cannot be assumed to be entirely harmlesss[11] One large Australian study showed that frequent ultrasound tended to restrict foetal growth. Another randomized controlled trial of 9,000 women in Finland found a slight increase in miscarriages after 16 weeks in those who had scans between 16 and 20 weeks.[12] A US study found a weekly scan doubled pre-term labour in women at risk of giving birth prematurely. It has been clearly indicated that ultrasound screening does not improve perinatal outcome.[13] On the contrary, studies showed early diagnosis of birth defects or growth problems had an adverse effect because babies got delivered pre-term.

Ultrasound heats the tissue and the amniotic fluid. Researchers say this can cause pockets of extremely high temperature gas to vibrate and collapse, which could lead to toxic reactions. Unborn babies are said to perceive scans as very loud or high-pitched frequencies because vibrations are produced in the amniotic fluid. We also don't really know enough about how it can affect the brain. A Norwegian study showed an increase in left-handedness,[14] which suggests that scans have an effect on neurological development. When ultrasound was introduced for foetal imaging in the 1960s, it was a device for high-risk conditions. It was rapidly developed without proper evaluation even though researchers warned that it should be kept under constant review and not used in the early pregnancy months. Today there are many different types of ultrasound but there is still inadequate research into the potential long-term effects. Many experts recommend reducing the number of scans and to use them only if medically indicated.

## Doc's Advice

*During my pregnancies, I declined all ultrasound and Doppler tests, deferring instead to the old-fashioned obstetric stethoscope which meant my midwife could hear my baby's heartbeat by my 20th week – late by modern standards!*

*If you are having an ultrasound, consider the following:*

- *Use ultrasound sparingly, avoid unnecessary scans*
- *Minimize use of ultrasound before 20 weeks of pregnancy. The most sensitive time for development of brains defects is between 10 and 17 weeks of gestation.*
- *Work with an experienced ultrasonographer at a reputable site*
- *Use a scan machine that provides the least exposure in the shortest amount of time.*

DR LAUREN FEDER WHO HAD HER CHILDREN AT 34 AND 38

## COMBINED SCREENING

The optional, non-invasive procedures combine a maternal blood test with an ultrasound evaluation of the foetus, to identify the risk of chromosomal abnormalities such as Down's syndrome, genetic heart defects or spina bifida.

The advantage of *First Trimester Combined Screening* is that it's performed in early pregnancy, between 11 and 14 weeks. The fast results can help you decide whether you want to undergo further diagnosis. The hormonal levels in your blood are analysed and a scan is performed to measure the fluid in the back of the baby's neck. These figures are combined with your age to provide a risk assessment for genetic disorders.

The disadvantage is that you won't get a definite diagnosis. The results can be ambiguous and are never as accurate as more invasive tests such as the amniocentesis. You will get a statistical likelihood of having a baby with a birth defect. This is relative to your age, so increased age is not going to improve your result. Depending on the programme used, anything higher than 1:150 is classified as a positive or abnormal result.

You can integrate the results from the *First Trimester Combined Screening* with a second blood test, which is taken between weeks 14 and 18. This *Triple Test* or *Integrated Screening* is a little more effective because it's using information from the first and second trimesters of pregnancy. It's thought that about 90 per cent of Down's syndrome cases are detected with this test. But the results also leave you with a statistical likelihood rather than a specific diagnosis.

There is a further blood test available during weeks 15 to 20. Similar to the other tests, the *Quad Screening* measures the levels of three to four substances in the mother's blood. High levels of certain hormones and alpha-fetoprotein (AFP) indicate a higher risk for a neural tube defect. The main disadvantage is that only 2–4 per cent of abnormally high results go on proving to be a problem. This means that 96 to 98 per cent of women are put under a lot of stress for no real reason.

## Ambiguous Results

If the screening results are good – which they are in the great majority of cases – then massive relief follows. You have the medical *permission* to enjoy your pregnancy and can rule out more invasive diagnostic tests. But any reassurance or bad news comes in the form of cold figures and statistics which are open to interpretation and a certain amount of speculation. There are many *false positives* where it seems like there's a problem when in effect there isn't one. Bang goes the reassurance you were hoping for. Instead you're left worrying even more and put under the kind of stress you were intending to avoid.

'When I had my first child at 39, my screening results were marginal. So at 43 I knew my chances of a bad result were even higher. But it's all based on computer programmes and they're not comparing you with other 43-year-olds. I researched it a lot and ended up going to a different clinic that used another system. My doctor phoned telling me I had a 1 in 30 chance of abnormality, so I panicked and booked an appointment for an amnio. But then realized I couldn't have an abortion anyway. In the end my actual screening result was 1:273; my doctor had overreacted. The whole thing was so stressful; it was all figures and eventualities and my fault for being so old. And because I had waited so long it was now my responsibility to decide over life and death.'

MONIKA, HEALTHY BABIES AT 39 AND 44

If you get a bad result from a non-invasive screen, then deciding to terminate the pregnancy would mean you're risking aborting a healthy child. You still have the option of seeking out a more exact diagnosis with further blood tests, scans or more invasive diagnostic tests. However, do you know what you'd do with that knowledge? If it's taken a long time to get pregnant or you've had fertility treatment, you may not want to lose the pregnancy under any circumstances. Maybe you're not in a position to care for a child with birth defects and you'd rather not take any risks. Many of us are unsure what consequences a bad test result will have, and postpone the decision until we're confronted with the relevant news.

'I don't like surprises so I did the tests. I would never have aborted the baby, even if she'd been diagnosed with Down. I just wanted to know ahead of time so I could prepare for the eventualities.'

DORRIT, HEALTHY BABY AT 38

Most practitioners will advise a woman over 35 to go for these non-invasive tests. It's important to remember that the probability of having abnormal results is very small. And, of the unfortunate women who get a so-called positive (i.e. bad) result, a whopping 90 per cent end up having a healthy baby.[15]

'I had the triple test and it came back positive for Down's syndrome; it was very high. Luckily my partner Michael was just so certain, so I tried to put it out of my mind, but the moment she was born I was in a panic trying to get someone to tell me if she was Down. The staff obviously had no idea why I was panicking as she was fine, but it's one of the reasons I didn't have any more kids.'

CLAIRE, HEALTHY BABY AT 36

## CHORIONIC VILLUS SAMPLING (CVS)

Chorionic Villus Sampling (CVS) is an invasive pre-natal diagnosis that involves getting a sample of the placental tissue and testing it for genetic disorders. It's used to detect Down's syndrome, Tay-Sachs, cystic fibrosis and sickle cell anaemia. CVS won't give you a result for anatomical or neural tube defects.

Using ultrasound to locate the placenta, a cell sample is taken via the vagina and cervix. Alternatively a needle can be inserted into the belly in order to snip or suction off the sample. Both procedures take about 30 minutes and can be uncomfortable.

The main advantage is that CVS is performed between the 11th and 14th week of pregnancy, which is earlier than amniocentesis. Test results usually take one to two weeks and are quite accurate.

The biggest risk is the chance of miscarriage, which is around 2 per cent. Most people weigh up the pros and cons and decide only to test if their screening result is higher than the miscarriage risk (some would call this gambling). There's an added risk of infection, vaginal bleeding and amniotic fluid leakage, so it's worth making sure the prodder has a good safety record. It's also important that you rest adequately before and especially afterwards.

'I had an amnio at 40 and it was very traumatic because the doctor was young and inexperienced. She tried it three or four

times and I was shaking. She finally got it and told me to go home
and have a big glass of wine. I felt angry because I was providing
valuable training. She's probably quite good at it by now. The
next pregnancy I had a CVS and it was a doctor who'd done it
many times but he was showing another colleague, so I felt like a
specimen. It's tricky because there's a danger of nipping a toe or
finger with the needle. The doctor told me I'd bleed a bit. I went
home and proceeded to have a period. I phoned him and asked,
"Will I miscarry?" His answer was, "You might still be OK." I bled
for three days. You have to ask yourself if it's worth it.'

BETHANY, HEALTHY BABIES AT 40 AND 42

## AMNIOCENTESIS

Amniocentesis, generally called an amnio for short, is the most
common invasive test available and most frequently used by
women over 35. Many choose to have amnios but then change
their minds when they start feeling more pregnant and the baby
moving. Anecdotal evidence suggests that leaping off the treatment
table at the last minute is not uncommon.

Seen as a breakthrough in ante-natal diagnosis, it can provide a
lot of information about the baby's genes and its current condition.
A small amount of amniotic fluid, containing foetal tissues, is
extracted from the sac surrounding the foetus and the DNA is
examined for genetic abnormalities.

As for CVS, you lie on your back while the practitioner uses
ultrasound to locate your placenta and the foetus. You can have
your belly anaesthetized but because this injection may hurt many
women opt to go straight for the big prick (absolutely no pun
intended!). A long, hollow needle is inserted into your abdomen
to withdraw some of the fluid surrounding the baby in the womb.
The whole thing is usually over within half an hour.

The advantage of amniocentesis is that it's the most accurate
test available for chromosomal disorders; it's more than 99 per cent

likely to detect Down's syndrome. However, it does not detect all birth defects such as structural or developmental problems. The worrying doesn't necessarily end with a good test result and it won't take the uncertainty out of life.

> *'You can't take age into the high-risk bracket. Every woman, no matter how old she is, runs the risk of having a sick child. Down's syndrome is just one disease but there are a million other things you can't screen for. There is never a 100 per cent guarantee.'*
> CORINNA, MIDWIFE

Amnios are generally performed mid-second trimester, between weeks 15 and 18. Sometimes amnios can be done earlier but they're more risky due to there being less amniotic fluid. Samples are cultured in a lab so it can take a further one to three weeks to get the results. This means that if there's a problem and you decide to terminate, you would have a late abortion which is physically and emotionally trickier. An amnio is meant to be safer than CVS, although some sources still quote the miscarriage rate at about 1 per cent. Mild cramping, bleeding or amniotic leakage can occur so it's important to take it easy and try to rest a few days after the test. It's also recommended to drink more water starting a week before the test, because dehydration can affect the amount of amniotic fluid you have. Babies probably don't like the procedure very much and have been shown on scans to 'get angry' or move out of the way of the needle.

## POSITIVE TEST RESULTS

What a warped world we live in where a positive result is actually not the answer you were hoping for. If you get a positive result from a diagnostic test such as the CVS or amnio, then there are still some variables. First of all, you could decide to have a repeat test to confirm the result. Not all chromosomal patterns are easy to interpret, and lab errors do occur. A lot depends on the diagnosis you receive; some conditions have treatment possibilities and frequently 'minor' defects such as extra, missing or twisted chromosomes don't develop into problems. It's often assumed that a foetus found to be abnormal will be aborted. There may even be subtle pressure to do so. Taking time to make up your mind will save any regrets you could have later on.

Knowing that you're carrying an imperfect foetus can trigger conflicting emotions. You may feel shock, alienation and anger. At the same time you might feel very maternal about caring for this particularly vulnerable baby.

Deciding which disabilities make life worth living are beyond anyone's capacity. You can only really judge whether the demands will be too much on you as a parent and whether you can make this commitment. Spending time with a disabled person who has the diagnosed disability of your baby might help you get a clearer picture. At the very least it will show you the sacrifices and rewards involved. Family members will be able to give you an idea of the kind of attachment they feel, as well as the financial and emotional obstacles.

## Down's Syndrome

Down's syndrome is the most common chromosomal disorder. A positive result means your child is likely to suffer from mental and physical problems. An amnio can only detect the presence of Trisomy 21, it will not be able to tell you how severely retarded your baby will be. Some people with Down's syndrome have serious health problems but many go on to enjoy fulfilled, long lives and they are capable of extraordinary acts. If your result shows up positive for Down's syndrome it's worth researching what this actually means, and getting in touch with families or support groups of those living with it.

## *Trisomy*

Some forms of Trisomy are more severe. Trisomy 13 and Trisomy 18 are known to cause a baby to die shortly after birth. Because it is impossible to foresee exactly how devastating a birth defect will be, you cannot know how long the child will live or how much it will suffer. What is more ethical, giving a baby a chance to live or saving it from pain? These are some of the hardest choices to make as a parent and they don't come with clear answers.

## ABORTION

For those who have made the decision to terminate, the next hurdle is to see through the procedure. Having an abortion is not easy under any circumstances, but if it means the loss of a much wanted child it's truly heartbreaking. It can take a long time to come to terms with the feelings of guilt and remorse.

Abortion procedures vary but generally in the first 12 weeks of pregnancy a suction-aspiration technique is used which does not require cervical dilation. From 15 to 26 weeks, the cervix has to be stretched in order to empty the uterus using surgical instruments and suction. This is generally called dilation and evacuation. After the foetus is 24–25 weeks old it could theoretically survive outside the womb, so this raises ethical and legal concerns. Abortions after 26 weeks are very rare and linked to severe foetal abnormalities or where the life of the mother is threatened.

Legal issues surrounding abortion are different in every country, and there are few subjects that cause as much public controversy. If you ever end up having the pro-life/pro-choice debate with friends, their strong opinions might surprise you. It's a very personal and highly charged issue.

# CHAPTER 7

## Pregnancy – The Middle Trimester

### BABY

*Month 5, Week 17*

As big as your palm, the baby's crown-to-rump length is between 11 and 13 cm, weighing in at 100–150 g already. Its brain cells are multiplying at 25,000 times per minute and baby body fat is beginning to form. The foetal heartbeat is about twice as fast as your own, at 140–150 beats per minute.

*Month 5, Week 18*

The rapid foetal growth is beginning to slow down a little now as it reaches 12.5–14 cm and weighs around 150 g. The baby is getting nutrients and oxygen from your placenta via the umbilical cord; these two systems are connected but completely separate from each other.

## Month 5, Week 19

The baby is now around 200 g and 15 cm long and the nervous system is developing further. It can hear noises and react to sound; it can also perceive light and darkness.

## Month 5, Week 20

Now 14–17 cm long and roughly 260–280 g heavy, the baby is able to kick, turn, twist and punch actively in the womb, because there is still the space (for another 6 weeks or so). Its skin is protected from the surrounding amniotic fluid by a greasy, white coating called *vernix caseosa*. This coating is produced by glands in its own skin.

## Month 6, Week 21

Grown again – arms and legs are in proportion now and crown-to-rump the baby measures about 18 cm. The baby weighs around 300 g and is swallowing, digesting and excreting amniotic fluid; studies show that a foetus drinks about 500 ml of amniotic fluid in 24 hours.

## Month 6, Week 22

The baby is about half the length it will be at birth: 19 cm. It weighs about 350 g. The fingernails, eyelids and eyebrows can be clearly seen. Taste-buds are forming on its tongue.

## Month 6, Week 23

The baby is really starting to put on weight, at around 450 g and 20 cm long; its body appears a bit rounder. The skin is still translucent so you can see the veins, organs and bones, until all the fat deposits are made. The neurons are fully connected to the muscles, and brainwave patterns are said to be similar to those after birth.

## Month 6, Week 24

The baby is now 21cm and between 540 and 680 g thanks to more baby fat and growing organs, bones and muscle. The baby's face won't change much more now until it is born; it has eyebrows, eyelashes and hair on its head (those who aren't born bald).

## Month 7, Week 25

Your baby is now about 22–23 cm and 600–700 g. Its capillaries are filling with blood and vocal cords are working, so you might feel it hiccupping soon. If your baby were born now, it would have a good chance of survival.

## Month 7, Week 26

Really fattening up, with some babies as heavy as 900 g; the norm is around 650–700 g and the crown-to-rump measurement around 23 cm. The baby has clear sleep-wake rhythms and you'll be able to tell when it's particularly active or sleeping. Its senses are developing well now; it can taste, smell, touch and hear. The eyelids are also beginning to open and close.

## Month 7, Week 27

From now onwards, the baby is measured from head to toe, rather than crown to rump. This new length adds about 10 cm, so instead of being 24 cm, little whippersnapper is now 34 cm long, weighing in at 750–900 g.

## *Month 7, Week 28*

The baby is now over 1 kg heavy and 35 cm long. Apart from its body getting fuller and rounder, the brain is growing with grooves and indentations; a complicated network of neuron connections is forming.

# ME

## *Pure Me Time*

The middle pregnancy months – when nausea and anxiety have usually passed – can be the easiest. It's when most women begin to look and feel pregnant and get really into it (hurry up, only two-thirds left!). Enjoy this remarkable time of your life. Like all good things it will pass and you'll look back wishing you'd made more of it.

If this is your first child you have even more of a reason to do WHATEVER takes your fancy. For a few months after birth, maybe even a few years, being independent and flexible (good reasons why you didn't become a mother earlier) will be more ... shall we say ... challenging.

---

### THINGS TO DO WHILE YOU STILL CAN

- Visit museums, art galleries, photo exhibitions, poncy restaurants and other places that require hushed tones and where you would receive dirty looks if accompanied by a minor.
- Talk on the phone for ages, paint your nails and eat some raw chocolate (simultaneously).
- Sit in a library, take an interesting book off the shelf and enjoy the SILENCE.
- Go swimming (ideally snorkelling in the sea) – the feeling of weightlessness is an incredible contrast to the new 'normal'.

- Book some beauty treatments, get your hair cut/done, spend a long time just getting pampered.
- Shop with a friend, take ages, be indecisive, try anything on, buy rubbish – basically act like a 20-something for the last time in your life.
- Go on a meditation or yoga retreat – two will benefit from this, you won't ever get such a bargain again.
- Lie in on the weekends (and weekdays if you can), read the paper in bed, preferably the Sunday paper – all of it.
- Go to the cinema as much as you can; see all the films on your 'must watch' list.
- Spend hours just pottering around your home. If you do nothing in particular, that's great. Motherhood will require more efficiency and less time doing nada.

Now, this is a really good time to go away on holiday. Believe me, the perfect time. Go away with your partner, a friend or by yourself. Ideally, you can afford to go somewhere exotic, sunny and faraway, but Bognor Regis will also do, as long as you don't have to camp. You might have to leave that Machu Picchu excursion for another time, because if you're not used to the altitude, walking above 2,000 meters is not very comfortable. Choosing a destination where you can be relaxed and happy will have a positive effect on the baby and its development – it has been proven. And never again will it be so easy to travel with kin; they're so compact, quiet and well looked after by that nanny-in-utero.

## TRAVELLING WITH A
## LOW-MAINTENANCE COMPANION

- Take snacks for the journey; prepare sandwiches or a packed lunch if it's a longer trip.
- If you're flying long-distance, it's worth wearing support tights and drinking masses of water – even if this means

disturbing your neighbour every 5 minutes – ideally drink more before and after the flight.

- Walk around on the plane to avoid cramp.
- Take a bag with wheels – hopefully you won't have to carry your own case but there are always those moments ('You packed all that stuff, you carry it!'). Hand baggage with wheels is useful for those long airport corridors.
- Pack comfortable, light clothes that don't crease and can be washed easily. Washing clothes on holiday means you can take less (and you always wear the same few things anyway).
- Take your medical records with you, just in case you need them.

**ONCE YOU GET THERE:**

- Make sure you continue eating and drinking regularly, especially if it's hot. Take advantage of the local fresh fruit (peel it, if in doubt).
- Do some barefoot walking to get vitamin D from the sun and negative ions from the earth – this *grounding* neutralizes the harmful positive ions we get from mobile phones and computers.
- If you're somewhere quiet like a beach or in the countryside, take long walks and sing to yourself and your baby (providing entertainment for the local cattle).

## How Your Life Affects the Baby's

Our first 9 months have the ability to shape the rest of our lives. Genes give the blueprint of possibilities, but what really controls our fate is the environment we grow in. This is what scientists and researchers in the fields of cell biology, foetal origins and primal health research are discovering.[1] The intrauterine environment in which cells are formed plays a key role for physical and mental health, behavioural characteristics, temperament and even intelligence. Because a foetus is constantly learning and adapting to the world it will soon enter, its cells begin the process of adjusting inside the womb. Everything a pregnant mother experiences – the food she eats, the air she breathes, the thoughts she thinks and the emotions she feels – has an impact on the development of her unborn child.

Mother and foetus are in constant dialogue with each other via the placenta and umbilical cord. Each physiological change in the mother is communicated via hormones in the bloodstream to the baby. This influences the foetal nerves, hormones and immune system. Mothers also communicate subconsciously with their unborn babies and vice versa. Tests have shown that behaviour is spontaneously coordinated and that mother and foetus sleep and dream together. If a pregnant woman listens to a baby crying on headphones, the foetal heartbeat rises. The heartbeat also rises if she only thinks about being upset. Calming music on headphones will calm down the foetal heartbeat.[2] This new frontier in science shows how we are perfectly prepared for the environment we're born into.

### SECOND TRIMESTER CHEER-ME-UPS

- You start to feel your baby move; there's nothing more exciting and life-affirming.
- You can push to the front of ladies' toilet queues, airport security checks and cafeteria line-ups. If anyone complains, simply smile, shrug and point to your belly.
- You have every right to get the last seat on the bus.
- You have every right to report anyone who questions this privilege.
- You get to wear your comfy yoga clothes long after class.
- No one will complain if you burp, fart or wolf down your food like a hungry builder.
- You will not be outlawed or sent to finishing school for unladylike behaviour (such as the above).
- In just over half a year your baby will have smiled at you for the first time. Now that's enough to melt the Queen of Narnia's heart.

## *Things to Consider Now*

How and where should I give birth? (Read Chapter 9 now, consider your options, make a decision, write a birth plan and remember it's not set in stone.)

Should I enrol in ante-natal classes? (See below.)

## *What about Those Pre-natal Classes?*

Whether you fancy doing this is really up to you; it's often a good idea if you're unsure about birth. The participants aren't all *woolly-jumper-Birkenstock* types, despite what your partner might say. Either way you'll get into it much quicker than him, sitting self-consciously on the floor for the first time since Kindergarten (tell him he'll get more material for *entertaining the mates* anecdotes than that trip to Butlins with your granny).

Check your local facilities; some good addresses are:

Active Birth, Birthlight, Bradley, Calm Birth, Gentle Birth, HypnoBirthing and Lamaze. Most will offer a weekend course or evening classes.

## NURTURE

### *Big Is Beautiful*

Many women worry about gaining too much weight when they're pregnant. But you know what? Pregnancy is a time of nurturing and surrender. Your body needs to expand. There's a little being in there (any associations with *Alien* are completely legitimate). Admittedly your waist will disappear. This is completely normal. And as miraculous as you may find this, you can and will return to your pre-pregnancy silhouette. The healthier you are during pregnancy, the easier it will be afterwards. Pigging out may feel good in the moment you're stuffing your face but don't we always regret it when the belly's bloated? Overeating is a major cause of toxicity in the body, so it's best to eat only 80 per cent of your capacity. A pregnant woman doesn't actually need more calories. After the fourth month it rises slightly but you still only need 200–300 calories extra – that's about three pieces of fruit.

## IF YOU HAVE A SWEET TOOTH

Sugar addicts, there is help at hand. Xylitol, a healing *glyconutrient*, is a low-glycaemic, low-calorie sweetener. It is 100 per cent natural and vegan, deriving from fruit and birch tree bark. It tastes and looks like sugar – so you can even bake your cakes and make desserts with it – but doesn't trigger an insulin release.

Honey is not a bad alternative to sugar for use in herbal teas because it contains disease-fighting antioxidants. However it is quite high in calories.

## *Brainy Babe*

The vital nutrients for foetal brain development are unsaturated long-chain fatty acids (EFAs or DHAs), particularly from the omega-3 chain. This is the most important thing to add to your pregnancy diet, alongside folic acid. DHA is found in cold-water fish (notably sardines), algae and seed oils (flax, hemp, perilla and chia). It's why pregnant women are told to eat oily fish twice a week. Fish from the start of the food chain such as sardines, anchovies, herring and the common mackerel are considered safer concerning mercury contamination. They're also the best in terms of omega 3, proteins and mineral content. If you're still worried then add some cilantro to your meal because the mercury content of fish can thus be largely nullified. If you're vegetarian (or can't stand fish) use the above mentioned seed oils and eat algae such as marine phytoplankton – the most nutrient-dense food on the planet – or take supplements with algal-based DHA. Fish actually get their DHA from algae.

## ALGAE AND SEAWEED

These simple organisms formed the basis of life on the planet as we know it, and they still support it. Sea vegetables are packed full of the minerals, proteins and nutrients that our bodies need to regenerate new cells and detox. They also help control the Earth's climate, because for every tonne of algae grown, over two tonnes of $CO_2$ are removed from the atmosphere and replaced by oxygen.

## Eat Sardines, Be Happy ... and Sing!

This phrase, coined by Dr Michel Odent, is also the title of an article he wrote on what the most important needs of a growing foetus are.[3] Scientific data shows that the stress hormone cortisol blocks the metabolic pathway of unsaturated fatty acids. A happy pregnant mother is more able to absorb and process the DHAs essential for the baby's development. Therefore singing is highly beneficial to the growth of the foetus. So keep on singing your mantras, pop songs, operettas ... dance, laugh, drum ... basically do anything that makes you ENJOY LIVING.

## FOODS TO AVOID DURING PREGNANCY

- Large amounts of eel, shark, swordfish, tuna, king mackerel and marlin, as they can contain higher levels of pollutants
- Raw fish that hasn't been frozen beforehand as it may contain parasites
- Undercooked meat (rare steaks, etc.) because you could get toxoplasma
- Too much liver or liver products as they contain retinol, which is linked to birth defects
- Runny egg yolks which may carry salmonella; cook eggs fully and you'll be fine
- Soft and mouldy cheeses such as Brie, Camembert, Stilton and goat's cheese because they may contain listeria, which can bring on miscarriage

## Foods to Cut Back On (Avoid Entirely If You Can)

*Caffeine*: More than 4 cups of coffee a day can lead to miscarriage. Caffeine has been proven to raise the baby's heartbeat and adrenalin levels much more than in adults; it also stays longer in its blood. Coffee and tea are bad for mum because caffeine dehydrates, draws calcium out of the body and blocks iron absorption.

*Alcohol*: Every sip you drink goes straight into your baby's system in the same proportions. Some women continue drinking a bit of wine throughout pregnancy, but new research suggests it's best to cut out alcohol entirely.

*Refined carbohydrates*: White bread, white rice, refined cereals, cakes and biscuits.

*Refined sugar*: It's just giving you empty calories, raising your insulin and compromising your immune system.

*Saturated or hydrogenated fats*: Most of the processed oils found in supermarkets; go for cold-pressed oils instead and avoid fried food.

*Low-fat foods*: They are loaded with chemical additives and flavourings.

*Flavour enhancers*: MSG (monosodium glutamate) and preservatives such as sodium nitrate.

*High-fructose corn syrup*: Found in jams, soft drinks, baked goods but also soups, pasta sauces, cereals, etc. Linked to diabetes, obesity and found to contain mercury.

*Artificial sweeteners aspartame and saccharin*: These neurotoxins destroy DNA and are linked to brain tumours, chronic disease and infertility; also shown to be eliminated very slowly in foetal tissue. A Danish study of nearly 60,000 pregnant women found those who drank one diet soda a day had a 38 per cent higher risk of pre-term babies. With four diet drinks, this rose to a 78 per cent risk.[4]

To underline this, when I was pregnant with my son I was working at a writing assignment at closed-door meetings of the World Economic Forum in Davos. At one particularly high-level get-together, a senior medical scientist and well-known Yale professor volunteered some personal advice as we left the building: 'Just don't drink soft drinks when you're pregnant.' Loud and clear. Do read the labels to make sure what you're buying. Unfortunately this might mean spending two hours in the supermarket and coming out with three items. Don't worry too much; if you drink the occasional diet soda you won't harm your baby, but repeated consumption of these goods can cause problems. Please also check the next chapter for all the wonder foods you CAN (and should) eat.

## WHEN SINNING ISN'T SCORNED UPON

If there's one time people will understand why you absolutely need to eat that ice-cream before you get to the checkout, then it's pregnancy. If you must have tortilla chips at 3 a.m., go for it, it's better than having insomnia. Pregnancy is a time of letting go and enjoying your impulses. In fact – and here's some pleasant news after I bombarded you with warnings – eating CHOCOLATE when you're pregnant is GOOD FOR YOU. It's shown to decrease the risk of hypertension and pre-eclampsia, especially chocolate made from real cacao. And, as we all know, chocolate makes you happy ☺.

## STRETCH

### Yogi Mummy II

The second trimester is the ideal time to work on your strength and vitality. Many people find them teeth-clenchingly strenuous, but squats are particularly good for building strength safely during pregnancy (it's also a position you might end up in a lot during the birth). Learn to do different variations of postures to accommodate your changing shape and avoid compression of the uterus. You are literally *making space* for your baby. Cat, Cow and Child's Pose are all very good to alleviate the most common pregnancy complaint – lower back pain.

Weeing becomes a big issue when you've got a little emperor using your bladder as a throne. Pelvic control is vital if you want to avoid further incontinence and *accidents* while sneezing. Sucking in and letting go of your pelvic muscles – or *mula banda* as the yogis call it – is an exercise you can do anywhere, even secretly while you're going home on the bus. Just tense the muscles around your vagina and anus; hold for some seconds and then release. Repeat as often as you like; the more regularly you practise, the better you'll get.

> *'We talk about pelvic floor education. It's not about strengthening the pelvis, because you don't want the muscles to be rock hard. You need to know how to engage and release them for birth. It's about stability and control of breath.'*
>
> LYNNE ROBINSON, PILATES MENTOR

## PILATES

Pilates is a low-impact form of exercise that strengthens your core. It's important to join a pregnancy Pilates class or get an instructor to show you what's different.

By the middle trimester most women really enjoy doing pregnancy yoga. Remember that if you're in full-time employment you're entitled to paid time off work to attend ante-natal yoga classes (need any more encouragement than that?). For many women it's the ONLY time out from their busy schedules where they can lie down, breathe and enjoy what's actually happening to them. It gives you a chance to focus on yourself, your new role and your baby. Yoga also enables you to bond with bambino and it has a calming effect on both of you. Be aware that you're doing yoga and breathing for two.

> 'Having quiet time three times a week just focusing on my
> wellbeing and the baby's had benefits beyond belief. I found
> it so relaxing and it I felt like I was really preparing my body;
> strengthening and lengthening physically and psychologically. It was
> really empowering and made birth a less painful and frightening
> experience.'
>
> JAZZ, BABY AT 38

Apart from bonding with junior, ante-natal classes are a good way to meet and connect with other women who look and feel *just like you*. Relating and sharing information has helped many a woman in need; often co-yogi-mums become friends for life.

## RELAX

### *Mantra Mum*

The middle months are a lovely time for singing mantras, as the foetus can hear from about 16 weeks, so apart from being relaxing for mum they're blissfully calming for baby. A mantra is like a sonic massage for your in-utero cub because he can feel as well as hear sound. It's also proven that after they're born, babies recognize the voices, sounds and music they heard in the womb. This makes singing mantras a great mothering tool for you to use postnatally, to soothe your child.

Sanskrit mantras connect us back to the source of sound. Sanskrit is believed to be a sacred language because it was conceived at the beginning of civilization when sages had revelations about the cosmos. The sounds make the palate vibrate in a certain way, affecting specific areas of the brain. The pituitary gland in our brain vibrates at the same frequency as the sound in order to harmonize with it. Apart from creating a soothing, trancelike state, it's a healing, complete body experience because all the cells in your body have the ability to vibrate at the same frequency as the sacred sound. This phenomenon can be observed in all religious chanting, praying and drumming. In Sanskrit, the original sound or mantra is simply, 'Aum' or 'Ohm', which is often chanted at the beginning and end of yoga classes.

A good pregnancy mantra is one that is passed down from all mothers to their children in India: the Gayatri mantra. It's a wonderful lullaby to sing before and after birth. You can also find soothing recordings of it:

> *Om bhur bhuvah svah*
> *Tat savitur varenyam*
> *Bhargo devasya dhimahi*
> *Dhiyo yo nah prachodayat*

## GLOW

### Pamper that Mama

Pregnant ladies love to lather up in oils and creams. Partly because it feels good to rub all those new, rounder bits but also because moisturizing the skin can increase elasticity. Nobody wants stretch marks, so we try to avoid these as best we can – ideally by putting on weight gradually – but if that fails we can try 'rubbing them out'. Plant-based essential oils penetrate the deeper layers and allow the skin to breath: jojoba, avocado, sesame, wheat germ, almond and olive oil all work equally well. Smearing expensive anti-stretch mark creams onto your belly won't do a better job, and paraffin-based creams will just stay on the surface of the skin.

Pregnant skin is not always glowing; sometimes it's itchy, swollen and blotchy. About half to three-quarters of all women develop hyper-pigmentation when they're expecting. If you're dark-skinned you get light blotches and if you're light-skinned you get dark blotches (nice!). Chloasma, also known as the 'mask of pregnancy', occurs mainly in the face (the most inconspicuous place, of course) and it's aggravated by sunlight. Rather than staying indoors with zinc block covering your entire body, opt for the Michael Jackson look: hat, sunglasses (OK you can omit the scarf over the mouth) and try to stay under the shade of a cooling tree or big person. Herbalists recommend using an infusion of daisy (2–4 g per cup of water) dabbed on the skin. You can also try aloe vera gel or rubbing pieces of red onion over the affected area (then ask if anyone fancies a kiss). Chloasma usually goes away entirely after childbirth.

## Belly Shopping

By the second trimester, with your improvisation skills exhausted, it's the perfect time to introduce some new guests to the wardrobe. Don't let your change in body image trigger a crisis; see it instead as an excuse to go shopping (physically or online). Yeah, shopping! Now, how come that word has lost some of its appeal? Maybe your priorities are shifting already?

The key to maternity wear is 'less is more'. You don't need to buy half the collection because chances are you'll wear the same few items over and over again. Also you may not (want to) believe it now, but you will get bigger still, and in some places more than others – that booty, for example. The key is to purchase a few essentials so you can layer your look and shed clothing as your temperature fluctuates. A couple of t-shirts and vests are useful; pregnancy ones are cut longer to cover your bump, and some of them have extra breast support. Cardigans and jackets are ideal because they open at the front for ventilation (very handy later, too, for breastfeeding). Trousers that expand at the waist are not just comfortable but they do actually look good, once you put a top on. A wrap dress can look great and if you need a glam evening frock you can go for a floor-scraping gown à la Hollywood. If it's winter you can probably get away with wearing your coat open and draping a thick, warm scarf in front, rather than forking out on a new coat you'll wear for only 3 months. For summer bunnies and swimmers there are some flattering maternity two-piece swimsuits with long tops that cover your middle.

As for materials, go for natural fabrics such as cotton, because acrylics can make you get very hot and sweaty. Also, your skin can become quite sensitive during pregnancy. The last thing you want is a scratchy, synthetic fibre irritating it more. Soft, stretchy jersey material is also good because it grows and moves with you.

Your retail therapy might involve indulging in shoes. However, chances are your feet are quite swollen now, and will continue to swell with your bump, so these shoes will not fit after you've had the baby. Another thing to consider is that feet often grow one size during pregnancy – and they STAY bigger afterwards, so wait and you might have to replace ALL your shoes anyway.

If you're completely broke or just can't be bothered with it all, ask your friends. Many of them will be happy to pass on maternity clothes they only wore once or twice.

## LOVE

### Engorgement All Areas

The second trimester really is the best part when it comes to your wellbeing, and it's thus also the sexiest. Uncomfortable side effects like sickness have usually worn off. You feel energetic and elated, like a buoyant schoolgirl at the start of the big summer holidays. And then there's that body: that gorgeous, juicy, ripe body.

I have mentioned breasts before, but I have to mention them again because they are practically worth getting pregnant for. Almost everybody loves enlarged, gravity-defying boobs. Our visually fixated society is obsessed with them. When I finally and proudly progressed up the cup-size alphabet was when I realized what the perfect (often silicon-filled) breasts are modelled on: an ample mammary bursting with milk. How primitive is that in terms of fulfilling original needs?

Speaking of which, pregnant women are known for having wildly erotic dreams. The kind where you have sex with strangers in different locations (your husband is mysteriously not there) and orgasm in your sleep – yes, you read correctly: you can actually physically orgasm without touching any floppy bits. Here's some more great news: increased blood supply to the uterus and pelvic area can heighten your sensations, making all acts of sex more enjoyable. It might be worth warning anyone about to perform oral sex that no, you're not turning into a baboon, thanks for the comparison, but those lovely pregnancy hormones have enlarged your genitals and changed their shade and taste. Yum! When (hopefully not if) you orgasm, the contractions or spasms are likely to be stronger, deeper and longer than the ones you had in your non-pregnant state. Did I say bigger boobs were the reason to get pregnant?

Unless you're particularly creatively endowed or know the Kama Sutra standing on your head (quite!) then the repertoire for intercourse starts to become a bit limited. Missionary style is out because you can't lie on your back any more, let alone have a 12-stone man jump around on your swollen belly, sore breasts and already compressed organs. The main three positions for pregnant sex are a) girl on top: perfect for both because you can determine the pace and he can admire the spectacular view of your heaving bosoms; b) doggy style: also works if penetration is not too deep, for extra comfort cushions, pillows and padding are the way to go; and c) spoon position (both lying on your sides): this is really comfy because no pressure is placed on the womb. However, the likelihood of you falling asleep may be bigger than either of you coming.

To really make the most of all this heightened activity in the sexual department, the middle months provide an ideal window for taking a trip – a kind of pregnancy honeymoon. This may, after all, be your last chance to enjoy time TOGETHER ALONE for a decade or two. If you're single or he can't take time off (and you don't want to file for divorce just yet) go away by yourself or with a girlfriend. Many of us females prefer shopping to sex anyway.

---

### THE SECOND TRIMESTER FOR HIM

It's sunk in: he's definitely going to be a dad soon. He starts to panic about the mortgage, his salary, the extension that needs doing, whether he'll be a crap dad, will you produce a monster? (Judging by your current behaviour, he thinks yes!)

He uses your pregnancy as an excuse to fart and snore again (you can't really tell him off now!) and he's pigging out as if it's a competition whose belly gets bigger. He cancels his gym subscription in order to *save up for the baby.*

He's so fascinated by your breasts he suggests repeating *this pregnancy thing* for seven more rounds.

---

## WORK

### Coming Out

If you haven't taken a holiday by the middle months you're probably desperately looking forward to precious time off. To be entitled to maternity leave you need to tell your boss by the end of the 15th week before your due date – that is around week 25 of your pregnancy, so actually in your third trimester.

This is a big moment in your relationship with your employer – similar to when you had to tell the headmistress that an important trip to see your great-aunt in Australia coincided with exams. It really helps to research and prepare well. If you think they may want to pull a dirty one on you, know the company's maternity-leave policy and your statutory rights (you can find all the latest details of maternity rights online, so I won't bore you with them here). It might be useful – and ever so impressive – to prepare a plan illustrating how you will wrap up work before you leave and in what capacity you plan to come back. This also gives you a chance to voice your ideas, needs and concerns.

### WAYS TO TELL YOUR BOSS

'I'm thrilled to announce that my current pregnancy will boost my performance at work and I'll come back committed to combining work with family life.'

'Something weird is happening. My tummy keeps getting bigger. I think I'm expecting.'

'You know that I treat every project like my baby. I'm now finally going to have one.'

'I've worked long and hard at this job. I'm definitely old enough. Everyone else has done it. Now it's my turn.'

'Can you give me some time off to birth a baby and breastfeed?'

'I have a bun in the oven. I don't know if I'll ever come back but I'll take the maternity leave and see how I feel.'

Once you've told your employer, they're not allowed to spill the beans to your colleagues or discriminate against you in any way. They're legally obliged to offer you regular periods of rest (stuff the staff report, pass the ice-cream and the remote control). They also have to give you a health and safety assessment (no more climbing up wobbly ladders to get dusty files from the top shelf). The hours must be reasonable (11 a.m. to 3 p.m., anyone?) and you're allowed to take time off for ante-natal appointments and – isn't this fantastic? – 'parentcraft and relaxation'. Women who work shifts, stand for long periods of time, do physically strenuous work or are exposed to potentially harmful chemicals can ask to be transferred.

## WORRY LESS

Even if you're feeling great, there might be a few annoyances that are completely new if you've never been pregnant before.

### Heartburn

This is a nuisance that doesn't go away for many women. Caused by the relaxing of the ring of muscle between the oesophagus and the stomach, harsh digestive juices travel back up the body, causing a burning sensation around the heart – hence the name! Eat small morsels of food slowly, chewing a lot more than you would normally (think of Daisy the cow). Avoid eating spicy, oily, sugary or acidic foods. Also steer clear of coffee, black tea and fizzy drinks (*quelle surprise!*). Try to avoid drinking at mealtimes as it stretches the stomach; it's better to drink some camomile or lemon balm tea about half an hour before. Pineapple and papaya are both good remedies for heartburn because they aid digestion; it is best to eat them in between meals rather than for dessert. Foods that can help neutralize stomach acid are cumin seeds, peeled almonds soaked overnight in water and wholegrain bread. If you get heartburn, particularly at night, use some extra pillows to elevate the top half of your body.

### Blood Pressure

High blood pressure, or hypertension, is not a cause for alarm unless it is accompanied by protein in the urine – which can be a sign of pre-eclampsia. The main way to avoid blood pressure complications is again through a good diet of fruit, veg, wholegrains, omega 3-rich foods, bananas and the algae spirulina. Studies show that acupuncture, aromatherapy and homeopathy can bring down raised blood pressure. Getting plenty of rest and staying well hydrated – in this case with dandelion tea due to its high calcium and potassium content – will ensure fiddle-fitness.

## TJM rather than TCM

**'If you find the thought of thick needles sticking into you off-putting, then you might prefer Japanese meridian therapy to traditional Chinese acupuncture. The needles are so thin in Japanese acupuncture you'll hardly feel them. It can be a more gentle treatment during pregnancy; you could also try Shiatsu and acupressure.'**

DR JONATHON DAO ND, OMD

## Water-retention

Swollen feet, ankles and legs are annoying pregnancy ailments mainly because it's not such a good look and your shoes don't fit. It's due to the hormone relaxin, which loosens the pelvis for childbirth, and can be aggravated by hot weather, fatigue and long periods of standing. Make sure you get plenty of exercise to keep blood and circulation pumping, as well as resting with your feet up. You can massage your ankles and feet with diluted geranium and cypress essential oils, or try hydrotherapy and lymph drainage. An Ayurvedic remedy is four parts boiling water with one part barley juice drunk as a tea; or try applying a 2:1 ratio turmeric-salt mixture to the area. Swelling does go away once you've had your baby, but as mentioned earlier many women find their feet stay one size bigger; never a better excuse to buy new shoes.

# CHAPTER 8

## Pregnancy – The Last Trimester

### BABY

*Month 8, Week 29*

Between 37 and 43 cm long and 1.25–1.3 kg in weight, the baby is due to double or even triple its weight before birth. Even though you now have more amniotic fluid in the womb, the baby starts filling it out, so sharp kicks may be replaced by knee, elbow and pointy bum pokes.

*Month 8, Week 30*

Weighing 1.35 kg and just a little longer than last week, your baby still has just about enough room in the womb to do a somersault. It's also starting to shed the soft body hair that has been keeping it well insulated.

## Month 8, Week 31

The baby has grown to about 40–46 cm and weighs around 1.6 kg. The skin on its face is becoming smoother thanks to all the extra baby fat it's accumulated. The good connection between nerves and muscles means it can coordinate its movements quite well now.

## Month 8, Week 32

Measuring 42 cm and weighing 1.8 kg, the baby's organs are all nearly formed; they just need to mature more before birth, especially the lungs. The intestines are filled with meconium: a thick dark-green mass of old cells, faeces and waste from the liver.

## Month 9, Week 33

Your baby is likely to be around 2 kg heavy and 43 cm long. Its skin is getting more and more rosy and its face smoother. For the growth of its bones it needs extra calcium and it's also taking antibodies from you, in order to develop its own immune system.

## Month 9, Week 34

Around 44 to 50 cm long and 2.3 kg heavy, the baby may already be in the position it needs to be for birth. Your placenta, which is providing the baby with food and oxygen, has developed all it needs to by week 34 and from now until birth it will just 'age'.

## Month 9, Week 35

The last weeks are all about putting on more weight before birth. The baby will weigh around 2.5 kg now and be 45–50 cm tall. Brain development is also a top priority. By this week the baby should have turned into its final position ready for birth.

## Month 9, Week 36

At 2.7 kg and 46–51 cm tall, the baby is more or less ready for life outside the womb. Its digestive, circulatory and other systems are well developed and it's actively producing the hormone cortisol in order to fully mature the lungs.

## Month 10, Week 37

If the baby – nearly 3 kg and around 50 cm tall – were to be born now, it would not be considered pre-term. Its lungs are fully developed and would be able to function well. The baby is producing hormones which will help determine on which day it's born.

## Month 10, Week 38

The weight and length of your baby will probably not change much more now. Around 3.1–3.6 kg and 47–51 cm, depending on whether it's a girl or a boy, are average this week. The baby will also shed the protective vernix coating and body hair ready for birth.

## Month 10, Week 39

It may be getting quite cramped in the womb and the baby's head could be dropping deeper into your pelvis, ready to push out. Its skull is soft so that the bones can slide into each other, protecting the brain on its journey through the birth canal.

## Month 10, Week 40

This is officially when your baby is full-term and may be born at any moment. However, don't worry if it's not happening yet. Around 50 per cent of babies are born after the due date. You should be given a good two weeks before the doctors start knocking at your door.

## ME

### Ballooning

Your little baby is not so teeny any more: it's starting to fill its first home rather well. It can be sitting right on top of your rectum so you may get pelvic pressure and backache. You also have more problems breathing, eating, peeing, walking and sleeping. Is it any wonder? – you're sharing your body with an extra person! Even if you're completely fed up and just dying to sleep on your tummy (or back) and finally see your feet again, remember *it ain't gonna last forever.*

Your bulge will attract the hands of strangers. If you don't feel like being groped, just say; 'Shhh, you'll wake the baby!' and walk off.

---

### SLEEPING COMFORTABLY

- Make sure you get enough exercise during the day: walking, yoga and swimming are the best during later pregnancy.
- Eat your dinner slowly a couple of hours before bed and if you're hungry again just take a light snack before going to sleep.
- Some relaxation exercises or a short meditation can help clear your mind. If thoughts are still bothering you in bed, keep a notepad handy and 'deposit' all the worries and 'things to do' there.
- Sleep in a well-aired, darkened room. Unplug all electrical devices.
- Pillows, pillows, pillows; you can never have enough during pregnancy – for under hips, belly, stray arms, knees – and

> you can also get one of those banana-shaped breastfeeding cushions.
> - Try putting a few drops of lavender oil on a hanky or use a small lavender sachet.
> - Sleeping on your left side might be the most comfortable and ensures an unobstructed blood-flow to all your organs and extremities.

## Baby Prepping

The last months get quite exciting; what with unfolding and refolding the teeniest, cutest baby garments to getting extra help by fit strangers when you're carrying heavy bags to the ultimate pre-natal party: the Baby Shower. Now this really *is* a fun day out (or in, if you make the mistake of having it in your home). It's a party where strictly women only are allowed – with the exception of any man-child offspring. A baby shower is celebrated to welcome new life into the world, but seeing as the pre-birthday child is still inside your tummy, it's really *all about you*. This gathering of goddesses will fill you with so much feminine power you could be high until well after the birth ... about until you get the baby blues. There are many ways to do it but the original rules were that your friends organize it and you give them a list of the things you need to ensure the presents are all useful and you don't end up with 15 white, size one baby grows. I've been to some pretty good baby showers – including my own beach baby shower – and always came away loving being female.

## Essential and Non-essential Baby Stuff

Admittedly some baby accessories are useful and were invented to make our lives easier. But we live in a very complex world with too much 'stuff' for our needs. This has nothing to do with the products greedy corporations want to flog from the overfilled shelves of shopping centres (and promote by evil means, taking advantage of our '*isn't that just tiny and adorable?* hormones'). Just because something exists, doesn't mean anyone actually has a need for it. And just because you can afford it, doesn't mean you have to buy it. A good rule of thumb is: forget anything that puts distance between you and your baby. Also, see what you can borrow or *inherit from* friends. Remember you will receive lots of gifts, so don't buy too many clothes, especially for under 3 months – they outgrow them SO fast. The shops will still be there after the baby is born; you can always buy stuff as you go along.

### Favourites

- **Newborn nappies** – and something to wipe poop off with like wet wipes or cotton wool
- **Newborn car seat** – the law, actually
- **Baby sling** – you may need this more than a pram in the first weeks
- **Baby clothes** – sleep suits, bodies, vests, socks, hat and some cardigans or jumpers with buttons for layering if it's cold
- **Soft blanket or wrap**
- **Soft towel**
- **Moses basket** or newborn cot – even if you're co-sleeping, this is useful for naps
- **Muslin squares** – there'll be constant wiping and mopping up, so get enough
- Some kind of **changing mat** – can also be a blanket on the floor
- **Nursing bra** and breast pads for leakages.

### Can Wait/Not Essential

- **A baby nest, mat or bouncy chair** so you can put the baby down somewhere while you shower
- **Pram** – this is an item you shouldn't impulse buy, so take your

time and try it out once you have a baby to push – see also Chapter 10

- **Baby bath** or non-slip mat for the big bath. I prefer the womb-like bucket type tubs, although you'll only use it for the first year or two. Some people just use the sink
- **Highchair** – your baby can't even sit for the first 6 months, let alone eat at a table, so this can wait
- **Cot or baby bed** – see how you get on with the sleeping arrangements and then get one to suit your needs
- **Breast pump** – might need it, might not
- **Baby monitor** – even if you live in Buckingham Palace, chances are you'll be close enough to hear your baby; most systems produce electro-smog
- **Baby hammock** or cradle – can be very soothing for them to be suspended and rocking
- **Nappy changing bag** – practical item to keep all the baby stuff neatly separated and fast to find in those baby-was-just-sick-all-over-everything emergencies.

## Matter of Taste/Money Thrown Away

- **Baby toiletries** – best not to use anything on their skin except water with maybe a few drops of almond oil in the bath. Babies don't sweat or stink. When they start crawling and do get grubby, I'd get all the organic stuff
- **Nappy disposer** – plastic rubbish
- **Baby walker** – more plastic rubbish with short shelflife; not so good for their joints to walk earlier than they're ready and is potentially dangerous for accident-prone kids
- **Bottle warmer and sterilizer** – some love them but most find they just take up space in the kitchen; boiling in a pan does the job just as well
- **Cot bumpers** – can be hazardous for a child under one due to the risk of suffocation

- **Playpen** – a baby cage that puts bars between you
- **Changing table** – an ordinary table or chest of drawers will do
- **Baby rucksack** – unless you're an avid hiker, a normal baby carrier is less bulky and does the job.

### LAST TRIMESTER CHEER-ME-UPS

- Becoming a mother will give your life a sense of meaning – even more than weekend trips to New York (well, almost).
- 'No frills' (what a term!) airlines let you board first without having to pay the extra tenner. You can continue taking advantage of this privilege after your child is born until it graduates (hey, you can try!).
- You will get Mother's Day cards – and, even better, Mother's Day presents.
- After you've been through childbirth, your partner will never call you a wuss again. If he even merely implies it, you can clobber him without being reported to the authorities.

## Choosing a Name and Other Last-minute Panics

Many people are clueless until the baby is born and they try on the name for size. It's good to have a few prepared but it's not worth getting your sexy pregnancy knickers in a twist over it. My partner and I just couldn't agree on a name. We practically broke up over it (I kid you not). From what I hear, this is a common problem and gives you a taste of the very heated differing opinions you'll have about *what's best* for your mutual offspring. It's really hard to agree. I personally think the woman should have the last word because she has to go through labour. But then my partner believes the contrary, of course. He reckoned because the woman has done everything else, the man should pick the name. Whatever! In the end we found a name we both liked the day before I went into labour. As most things in (married) life, you usually find a compromise where both of you believe you got your way (I agreed to his all-time favourite as a second name, so it wouldn't come up again next time round).

Another very useful thing to get your head around – if you can muster up the energy and creativity – is preparing and freezing meals for after the birth (remind your partner they're not for him while you're in hospital). You'll be so relieved when you're stuck home alone and your day is taken over by the baby's need for constant feeding. You may barely be able to shower or comb your hair, so the last thing you'll manage is to cook a decent meal. And remember, if you're breastfeeding, it makes you very, very hungry – to the point of gluttonous, sinful greed. So stock up on what you need, because shopping is not an easy task in the first weeks.

Also, wash some of the newborn clothes, because baby skin is very sensitive to the chemicals in clothes fresh off the rail. Keep some clothes with their receipts just in case you have a bigger baby who goes straight into the next size up.

### THINGS TO CONSIDER NOW

- If you haven't already planned your birth (well, some people like to be more spontaneous), now's the time to do so.
- Nursing bras that open for feeding – from around week 36 they should fit.
- How to communicate the birth – cards or virtual announcement? (We designed a simple website rather than sending out 15 hormonal photos all looking the same to clog up inboxes).
- Where your little Einstein will go to school (only joking, although some people really like to plan ahead).

## NURTURE

Towards the end of your pregnancy, a bigger baby is taking up the space where the stomach used to be, so you'll find that you get full very quickly. If you haven't already switched to six small meals rather than three big ones, do it now. Make sure you always carry fruit, nuts, seeds or light snacks for those *eat now or kill someone* moments.

### *Fab Foods for Pregnancy*

*Dates and figs* – blood-building, which is so vital in pregnancy.

*Bananas* – fast fix if your blood sugar level drops and provide fibre.

*Avocados* – vitamin E + $B_3$, folic acid, iron, potassium and monounsaturated fats.

*Almonds* – soak raw, unprocessed almonds overnight in water so they're easier to digest; they're rich in absorbable and high-quality protein, vitamin E and $B_2$.

*Seeds* – pumpkin, sunflower and flaxseeds are rich sources of omega 6 and omega 3, great to nibble on instead of sweets. One cup of sunflower seeds gives you nearly half your daily vitamins and over half your minerals.

*Sweet potatoes* – contain 60 minerals (white potatoes only have 3) also low glycaemic index which is great for sustained energy release.

*Broccoli* – just one cup covers a quarter of your daily vitamins; a folic acid veg.

*Celery* – folic acid and vitamin C, dip it in hummus or tahini for more flavour.

*Spinach* – packed full of calcium, magnesium, iron; eat it steamed or raw in salad.

*Quinoa* – the staple food of the Incas, quinoa is a protein-rich grain that is better than animal protein. It also helps you cope with stress and provides many B vitamins.

*Bulgur* – nutritious wholegrain rich in B vitamins, iron, fibre and protein that can be eaten warm or as a salad.

*Amaranth* – used by the Aztecs, this high-protein grain has three times more fibre content and five times more iron content than wheat; and twice as much calcium as milk. Also contains amino acids, minerals and vitamins. It tastes great as porridge.

*Oats* – B vitamins, good for digestion and sustained energy release.

*Lentils and chickpeas* – loaded with iron, phosphorous and calcium, these beans feed millions of vegetarians every day in India.

*Garlic* – good for healthy blood, great natural antibiotic and an antifungal vegetable.

## Superfoods

*Alfalfa* – highly nutritious plant that is loaded with magnesium, iron and calcium; also contains four times the vitamin C of citrus fruit, as well as digestive enzymes and amino acids.

*Blue-green algae* – contain every nutrient necessary for life.

*Bee pollen* – packed with amino acids, it also has 50 per cent more protein than beef.

*Spirulina and kelp* – Iodine, B vitamins, D, E and K and rich in amino acids.

*Sprouted seeds* – for the ultimate nutrition kick.

## JUICING FOR GOOD HEALTH

A wonderful way to get essential vitamins, minerals and hundreds of healing phytochemicals during pregnancy is by juicing fruit and vegetables. Juicing frees up the nutrients that are often trapped in the fibre of the food; this means they go straight into the bloodstream. You can add a sprinkling of your favourite superfood powder and, *hey presto!* all the goodness you need in one glass. For an instant health improvement make at least one green smoothie a day. Just mix green, leafy veg with a piece of fruit like an apple or banana.

## *Teeth and Bones*

It's recommended to increase calcium intake in the last trimester because the baby's bones are hardening and growing. There is a saying: 'With every child, you lose a tooth' – but it needn't be so if you watch your diet. Some doctors will encourage you to drink four glasses of milk daily to cover the extra needs but dairy is actually the worst source of calcium because it depletes the bones, partly due to its acidity. The countries with the highest dairy consumption – such as the USA and Finland – have the highest rates of osteoporosis. Humans are the only animals that drink milk after being weaned. Most adults find it hard to digest dairy and many are lactose intolerant. Milk products also elicit a high insulin response and are associated with childhood diabetes and certain autoimmune diseases. Fresh, raw milk from happy, grass-fed cows may be OK for some in small doses but the homogenized, pasteurized, highly-processed drink sold to us as 'milk' is full of antibiotics and other toxins; the same goes for most yoghurts and cheeses. It's preferable to get your calcium from foods such as green leafy vegetables, apples, cabbage, sweet peppers, sesame seeds, tahini, amaranth, edamame and black molasses.

## MATCHING COUPLE – IRON AND VITAMIN C

If you drink a glass of orange juice or eat a piece of fruit containing vitamin C before an iron-rich meal this will aid your body's absorption of the iron. Black tea and coffee can diminish the body's ability to absorb iron.

## Bistro Mama

If you eat out a lot you can still choose healthier food; go for a salad or soup for starters and pick a main that is steamed, grilled or poached. Eat at least a mouthful of raw food first, and take your own real salt with you rather than using what's in the shaker. You can ask for dishes with the sauce separately. If in doubt, ask for a lighter or healthier variation of something you fancy.

Before I let you off the hook about food (I know, I can be a pain, but be glad you don't have to live with me) I just want to introduce one more concept which may help your digestion and food absorption and is a great habit to set you up for life. Here goes (and I'll let someone else do the lecturing this time):

*'The stomach and digestive system are more sensitive during pregnancy so food combining is a good thing to practise. This will take the stress away from the spleen. A good functioning of the spleen is important because it is responsible for building blood to nourish the foetus. You can support the stomach and spleen through correct food combining and a balanced wholefoods diet. Eat cooked and raw foods according to the seasons and ensure you have an alkaline diet.'*

DR JONATHON DAO

## FOOD COMBINING

The theory goes: by eliminating the factors that obstruct your body to self-heal you can cure disease through diet. Also known as the Hay diet (as in William Hay), food combining says that you shouldn't eat proteins and carbohydrates together (a typical mistake would be steak and chips for example) because they require different conditions for digestion. Eat fruit around 30 minutes before or in between meals, because fruit is digested quickly. Hay also recommends that your diet contains four times more alkali than acid food, so that vegetables, salads and fruit make up the majority of what you eat.

Happy eating! Enjoy your yummy (mummy) food!

## STRETCH

### *Yogi Mummy III*

Towards the end of your pregnancy, yoga can help you feel more gracious and elegant rather than cumbersome and clumsy. Your sense of gravity may have shifted, but many heavily pregnant women are brilliant at balancing postures. It's all about connecting and being in harmony with the qualities of earth. Think about the secure, earthed support growing plants have, and how the trunk of a tree sustains and nurtures heavy branches. Yoga will also help you breathe more easily because the energy is not so compromised. It is all about flow – moving through stillness – and the rhythms of pregnancy fit perfectly with this.

Late pregnancy yoga introduces exercises to ease aches and pains. Pelvic girdle pain is a problem for many women but you can do postures to release this such as Cat and Dog against the wall. Classes have a special focus on relaxation and postures to open the hips and pelvis for birth. A lot of the exercises are now done in comfortable lying-down – sideways – positions with props such as cushions. You can also do an exercise to turn a breech baby, which is very simply lying with your legs up against the wall with your bottom slightly raised on a cushion. There are, incidentally, lots of other things you can try to turn a breech baby including acupuncture, reflexology and hypnotherapy. A remarkable study conducted in Arizona resulted in 81 out of 100 breech babies turning spontaneously after an average of four hours of hypnosis sessions; half of these turned after only one session.[1] Each mother (all were at least 36 weeks pregnant) was asked to talk to her baby to encourage it to turn, and visualize the uterus relaxing. In comparison, of 100 women who didn't have hypnotherapy, only 26 babies turned spontaneously.

Now is the ideal time to practise some good birthing positions because by the last months you're particularly interested in focusing on that big, inevitable, rapidly approaching event (definitely too late to back out now!). Surrender in yoga postures to become soft, supple and flexible. Embrace all that comes with a stillness of breath and a deep stillness inside – this may be the most important sensation to fall back on during the birth.

*'A woman's knowledge of pregnancy and giving birth is instinctual, and should be very empowering. The important point is to see yourself as a channel for a new spirit and to surrender yourself to all that the experience has to teach you.'*

DR CHRISTIANE NORTHRUP

By practising yoga, your body will have strengthened and toned – even if you can't see it right now. Thanks to yoga it should take you less time to regain your shape and fitness after birth, even all those hours spent in Corpse pose.

*'The birth of the baby is the beginning of another, much longer, journey of motherhood. Yoga practice can provide the best sense of continuity between pregnancy, birth and mothering. At every level – physical, mental and spiritual – yoga provides support through some of the most demanding and rewarding periods of a woman's life.'*

UMA DINSMORE-TULI[2]

## RELAX

*Visualize, Breathe, Affirm*

Our pregnancy pal, progesterone, has a very soothing and calming effect. You're probably less prone to fidgeting as your whole organism slows down, and you might find meditation easier as a result. This is a great moment to introduce some simple visualizations. These can involve picturing your baby floating happily in the womb or – if you're feeling brave – you can visualize the birth taking place, gently and naturally without any forced movements or excessive pain.

Another meditation you can do is to scan through the body and connect with each part. Hypnotherapists say it's very conducive to 'talk to' and 'thank' your internal organs for the big job they're doing in pregnancy. You can also 'visit' your baby, draw energy towards it and nurture it with light and love. Reassure it that the world is a loving, safe place and that you will protect and care for all its newborn needs; bond and build trust. By communicating thus with your baby you'll also be in touch with its energy and life force. After all, it's both of you who have to work together to get through the birth.

*'In the same way as your physical body is pervaded by the energy of your pranic body, so too is your baby; the baby's physical body is contained within your womb, but you are contained by the energy of the baby, as if the baby's prana is enveloping you.'*

UMA DINSMORE-TULI[3]

You can also try out some simple breathing techniques where you inhale and exhale through alternate nostrils. Use your thumb and ring finger to open and close alternate nostrils and hold your breath in between. Or you can simply breathe in deeply, hold your breath for as long as possible and then breathe out slowly. All these exercises are good for strengthening the lungs, improving circulation and flooding your system with oxygen. Meditation and breath awareness give you a reassuring, familiar place to go during contractions.

Because the mind–body connection is so powerful, positive affirmations are important tools to use throughout your pregnancy. Scientific evidence proves that babies in utero are tuned in to their mother's thoughts and feelings. You can meditate with affirmations, write them down, stick post-it notes with them around your environment, remember them when you're running for the bus and repeat them when you go to sleep at night.

By the last trimester, rather than feeling anxious about the birth, you can programme your body through the power of your emotions and thoughts. Spend a little time each day doing some simple birth affirmations and then let go. Trust your incredible body to do what it knows.

## GLOW

### *'Don't Touch the Hair!'*

During gestation you'll generally have many more good than bad hair days. Those previously lacklustre locks grow into a mane of thick shininess practically overnight. Some women do end up with limp, greasy hair, which is really unjust (who said pregnancy was just?). The big question many women ask is whether they can dye their hair. Chemical dyes are not particularly 'healthy' and they have been known to penetrate the scalp and cause allergies. If you want to continue staying 'autumn chestnut', rather than 'streaky grey' you can play it safe by using vegetable dyes and semi-permanent, ammonia-free colours. Getting highlights should be fine, providing the products don't touch your skin. Also remember hormones can make your hair react differently to the colour. It's definitely not a good time to get your hair permed or straightened because you could end up looking like Fuzzy Bear.

The downside to a healthy head of hair is a hairy body of hair. You may find hairs growing in previously smooth places such as chins and nipples. Plucking will get rid of the strays and waxing will keep the ape at bay. If you've never waxed before this could be painful as your skin is more sensitive during pregnancy. If you're feeling adventurous you could try threading. I get this done when I'm in India and always marvel at the skill of it. For those women who normally shave their fur, it's fine to carry on doing so. However, bleaching or using hair-removal creams is probably best avoided because of the chemicals.


## *Massage, Reflexology and Aromatherapy*

If there's ever a time when you could really do with a good pampering, then it's towards the end of pregnancy. A massage – by a therapist trained in ante-natal massage or a loving partner who knows what he's doing – can relieve insomnia, back pain and other aches. Research shows that women who are massaged during pregnancy have fewer premature babies, reduced anxiety and improved mood.[4] They also have fewer labour complications and less labour pain[5] (maybe one day when women rule the world, you'll be able to get them free on the NHS!)

You won't be able to lie on your derriere for a massage any more so a special table with a pouch for your belly is needed, or you can relax on your side supported by pillows. If using oils, go neutral or check the list below for essential oils you can mix with a base oil of almond, olive or wheatgerm oil.

Reflexology is the ancient art of accessing internal organs by massaging points on the feet. This can relieve aches and help your uterus relax. It's so powerful that it can bring on labour (so make sure your reflexologist is genuine). Studies show that reflexology gives outstanding pain-relief at birth. The results of Dr Motha's Gentle Birth Method 'The Jeyarani Way' showed that a course of ten reflexology treatments during pregnancy remarkably reduced the length of labour and the caesarean section rate in their client pool.

If you can't afford any spa treatments you can still create little oases of calm in your home to retreat to, with cushions, candles and music. Aromatherapy is one of the oldest forms of natural medicine, originating in ancient Egypt, India and Persia. The oils are easy to use; they can be inhaled or applied to the skin. Aromatherapy oils are strong, so make sure you're shown how to use them or follow instructions; usually it's about 10 drops of essential oil to 2 teaspoons of neutral oil such as cold-pressed olive, sunflower or almond oil.

### AROMATHERAPY OILS IDEAL FOR PREGNANCY

- **Chamomile** – natural anti-inflammatory and pain-reliever; good for backache, headaches, wind, constipation and nasal congestion
- **Lavender** – all-round oil, natural antiseptic and anti-depressant, it encourages cell renewal and relaxes muscles; good for backache, headaches, muscle and joint pain, insomnia, colds, stretch marks and infections
- **Geranium** – uplifting, balancing and pain-relieving, improves circulation and is anti-inflammatory; good for backache, swollen ankles and legs, colds and infections
- **Neroli** – anti-depressant, sedative and digestive; good for digestive problems (from constipation to diarrhoea), stress, anxiety and fear
- **Frankincense** – rejuvenating, anti-bacterial and comforting, good for stress, aches and stretch marks

You can also use coriander, cypress, ginger, grapefruit, jasmine, lemon, orange, pine, rose, sandalwood, tangerine and ylang ylang. *Oils to avoid during pregnancy* (unless you actually do want to trigger contractions): basil, hyssop, juniper, marjoram, myrrh, pennyroyal, peppermint, rosemary, sage, thyme.

## LOVE

### Touching Up

The final months are an important bonding time for soon-to-be parents with each other and the baby. Often us earth mums are so involved with our pregnancies that we forget to acknowledge our partners. Any high-maintenance men better get with it quick before the bomb drops in the form of a needy newborn. If you have the energy, give him some attention and include him in your baby caressing rituals.

Feeling the baby move is wonderful for you and even better for papa because it gives him a chance to get more involved. Encourage him in talking to his progeny through your belly; some men may feel stupid doing this but they'll warm up over time. Because babies can hear in the womb and will recognize voices once they are born, it's a good idea to get them familiar with yours. Even off-key, screechy singing will be a choir of angels to your newborn if it comes from his parents. Love is in abundance, so don't be afraid to wear it out.

There are great games you can play with a baby in utero. Endless hours of fun can be had rhythmically finger-tapping the bump and getting cheeky kicks in return. Or holding your hand against the belly and feeling a little, pointy bottom press against it.

### Intimate Threesome

Sex may not be the first thing on either of your minds right now. Interest and comfort generally wanes in proportion to expanding belly size. Your impressive cleavage is still growing but it has shrunk in relation to your bump. An added twist is that there are clearly now three in the bed. This is not the threesome your fella may have been dreaming about since puberty, it's merely the start of your sex life being destroyed by offspring. But just let's get the bigger picture here. A foetus tucked away in a dark corner of your womb is nothing compared to a dozing, angelic one-year-old lying on your side of the bed while you try hard not to get distracted (focus on penis! focus on penis!). Or how about a three-year-old poking his head around the door asking why daddy is squashing mummy (or vice versa if you're pregnant again).

## Well-endowed

Sex with a massively pregnant woman does raise a few interesting questions for the man. First of all, no, the baby's not listening (and if it is, it won't mind particularly). Secondly – and you gotta love this one – no, big he-man won't injure tiny baby. Your stud may confidently (or should we say arrogantly) think he's as well endowed as a porn star but there is no way he's anywhere near touching the baby because it's blissfully and safely immersed in amniotic fluid.

If you orgasm you're likely to have more spasms or so-called Braxton Hicks towards the end of your pregnancy. This is good. It's doubly good because it's preparing your body for labour and stimulating the uterus. Young sprog may even enjoy the free massage. If you're overdue then sex is to be encouraged because the prostaglandins in sperm can help soften the cervix and induce labour. However don't worry if you don't want to pop quite yet. Unless the cervix is ready, neither sperm nor spasms will bring on labour.

### THE THIRD TRIMESTER FOR HIM

- He starts looking at you with a mixture of pity and fear, especially when you step out of the shower.

- He's getting excited about having a new pal to play football with (in about ten years) and planning where they'll drink the first pint. If it's a girl he's already worried about the blokes who'll want to kiss her.
- Get ready for his softer, feminine side! In the first weeks after birth, new fathers see a rapid reduction in testosterone – the hormone that motivates them to mate, fight for status and take risks. It's nature's way of honing in on qualities more suitable to fatherhood.

## WORK

*Easy Now!*

When you're coming into the home stretch, everything is more of an effort and takes longer. Heaving that belly around packed trains and busy streets will make you wish you lived in the countryside (unless of course you do live in the countryside, then you might wish the shops were closer). Rather than taking it easier at work, you may be pushing yourself even harder in order to get things done before you go on leave. Planning a handover can also create extra work, so try to keep it as simple as possible.

During the last months, common late-pregnancy problems like backache, heartburn and breathlessness might make work a real pain to deal with.

### BACKACHE

If you're standing a lot, sit down regularly. If you're sitting a lot, make sure your chair is at the right height and supports your back. Use a cushion and a footrest. Have your work station assessed properly. Take regular walks, go to pre-natal yoga at least twice a week and swim. Indulge in massages.

If the last weeks are dragging on and the effort of going to work is too much, see if you can work from home or reduce your hours. If you can afford it and it's logistically possible you could ask for annual leave. Remember that if you're off sick in the four weeks prior to your due date, your employer can deduct this from your maternity leave.

On the other hand you could be bursting with energy, as many women are shortly before birth. The famous 'nesting instinct' might have you rushing around preparing your living quarters for the new permanent guest (is that a drill you're holding?). This is all well and good, but do remember to put your feet up between the activities. All the preparations will be cut short if you end up rushing to hospital because your waters broke while you were putting together that bloody IKEA shelf.

## WORRY LESS

Yes, it just gets better and better, doesn't it? As if that giant pumpkin attached to your waist weren't enough of a hassle you could have leg cramps, haemorrhoids, pregnancy diabetes or a vaginal infection. And you haven't even given birth yet. Oh boy!

### Leg Cramps

Most common at night and in the second half of pregnancy, cramps are caused by the extra weight you're carrying, circulatory changes or too little calcium and magnesium in the blood. When you get a cramp the best thing to do is stand up. You can also do stretching exercises such as upright wall press-ups before going to bed to try and keep them at bay. Also have a bath with lavender oil. Adding supplements or eating more calcium- and magnesium-rich foods may also help.

## Diabetes

Insulin is the hormone that regulates blood sugar levels. When there is a lack of insulin, blood sugar levels rise suddenly, causing diabetes. Pregnant women are more prone to getting diabetes because their blood sugar levels go up due to hormonal changes and they need to produce extra insulin to cope. Another reason is that the placenta produces hormones which block insulin production. If you're diagnosed you may be able to treat it by working together with a nutritionist to adjust your diet; cutting out sugar is obvious but sugar is hidden in so many products. Yoga can also help prevent and improve diabetes.

## Haemorrhoids

Painful, painful, painful, but unfortunately around half of all pregnant women get them. They are basically varicose veins up your bum after having serious constipation for too long and because that enlarged uterus is pressing down in all the wrong places. Lack of fibre and water in the diet, as well as insufficient exercise, are known culprits. Another way to prevent haemorrhoids is by doing your pelvic floor exercises regularly, because they increase blood flow and strengthen the pelvic wall and rectum. If you have them, ice packs can reduce pain and swelling. If they itch, a warm bath with camomile tea or witch hazel is soothing.

## Vaginal Infections

Thanks to all those lovely pregnancy hormones you're more prone to getting thrush or candida. Some doctors prescribe antibiotics but it is a vicious circle taking them. The usual over-the-counter remedies aren't really safe to use, so you need to go natural. You can also soak tampons in live yoghurt (preferably natural, not strawberry flavour) and insert them overnight. Cutting sugar and refined flour out of your diet and taking probiotics is known to help prevent getting thrush in the first place.

Another organism called Group B Streptococcus is often cultured in late pregnancy because there is a slight risk your baby can become infected during vaginal delivery – it is often treated with antibiotics. I was diagnosed with Strep B in the week before my due date (bingo!) and got rid of it by inserting garlic tampons up my vagina every night (just put a clove of garlic inside a sterile gauze and tie a knot). Yep, the smell isn't so great, but it worked.

## COUNTING DOWN

With birth around the corner you might suddenly have an overwhelming hormonal urge to change your birth plan entirely. If you can let the mammalian brain take charge, it's in fact a good thing because any other cerebral activity will just get in the way of the simple, animal task required of you now: getting that baby out. If you planned a hospital birth and decide you want to stay at home or vice versa, don't be afraid to voice your decision. Most healthcare providers should be flexible enough to accommodate your wishes and if you choose to birth outside of hospital this should be possible, providing your pregnancy has been uncomplicated. If you're suddenly afraid of the pain of childbirth, read the next chapter and think about your best options.

### PRE-TERM BIRTH

If your baby is born early, consider *Kangaroo care*. By keeping the baby skin-to-skin on you in a pouch continuously (or as often as possible) and exclusive breastfeeding, this technique has been shown to double the survival rate of pre-term babies, particularly those weighing less than a kilo. Studies found that half a million neonatal deaths could be avoided every year from London to Malawi by this low-cost intervention.[6] A parent's body temperature helps regulate the baby's temperature more smoothly than an incubator; plus, thanks to physical and psychological closeness, babies are shown to increase weight and strength faster.

## *Ready, Steady*

Having important numbers ready, enough petrol in your car, a clear idea of the best route to the hozzie – or enough old sheets and a full fridge if you're not planning on going anywhere – will help you to avoid panic in the crucial moment. If you're getting nervous, do your breathing exercises, relax and maybe think about turning to religion or something.

No matter what anyone tells you, it's UP TO YOU when you start packing your clinic case. My friend Laura had hers ready six weeks before the due date, whereas I waited until the last week – much to the annoyance of my mother-in-law, who had bought me fluffy slippers and a nightie so hideous I wouldn't even want to save it for the old folk's home (if this book is ever translated into Spanish, please edit this sentence out!). Those planning a home birth may think it's a bad omen to prepare anything, but I say forget superstition. Can you imagine looking for size zero bodies mid-contractions? This is the first time you'll have to pack for your baby. It's nearly as exciting as going on holiday.

---

**CLINIC BAG**

*For You*
- Snacks, CDs, oils, entertainment – anything you need for the birth
- An oversize, comfortable t-shirt or loose cotton dress to wear during labour
- Something to read (for those boring moments!?)
- Camera and charger (for after the birth rather than during, no matter how exhibitionistic you are)
- Mobile and charger
- Dressing gown
- Big, old knickers you were going to throw out or disposables (yep, they get pretty ruined) and big, fat sanitary towels
- Breast pads and breastfeeding bra

---

- Make-up bag
- Going home clothes

*For Your Baby*
- Newborn nappies and wipes
- Baby clothes (a couple of bodies, cardigans, your favourite newborn outfit, warm cap, cardigan, socks)
- Soft blanket – plus a thick one if it's cold
- Soft towel

Also, don't forget to have that car seat in place.

## If You're Overdue

- Don't start biting your nails.
- Tell all those people who keep calling that the doctor confused your due date and it's not actually for another two weeks.
- Relax. About half of all babies arrive overdue, and studies show that this is down to the date of conception not being clear.
- Go to the cinema; if you can't move from the sofa, order in and see some good films.
- Watch the moon and get in touch with your female, yin energy.
- Distract yourself by seeing friends (those who don't ask when the baby's due) and enjoy being ALONE – you won't have this privilege for the next 20 years.
- Overdue babies are hereditary (according to some Danish scientists), so blame your mother, father or both.
- Bounce up and down or drive over a bumpy road.
- Drink raspberry leaf tea.
- Empathize with elephants: they are pregnant for 20 to 23 months!
- Make some delicious food.

- Don't worry, you won't stay pregnant forever. Your little one just isn't quite ready yet. Latest studies show that the baby gives the impulse to start the birthing process.
- Start knitting, learn macramé.
- Eat some spicy curry.
- Have some acupuncture or reflexology.
- Eat some fresh pineapple.
- Go for long walks to help draw that baby into the pelvis.
- Have sex with ample nipple stimulation.
- Drink more raspberry leaf tea.
- Start biting your nails.
- Now try that castor oil cocktail your grandmother used ... (only joking!!).

If you are two weeks over your due date you should ask to have a scan to check how your baby is doing, whether there is still enough amniotic fluid and the condition of the placenta. This is, according to Dr Michel Odent, the most useful scan to have in pregnancy, but unfortunately the one least commonly practised.

### WHAT IF THEY WANT TO INDUCE?

It's easy to undermine a woman's confidence by saying there's an increased risk due to her age and that labour should be induced. Going from pregnancy to labour is a very delicate process, so the last thing you want is to worry; it's counterproductive to the hormones needed during birth. Induction can result in birthing a baby that isn't ready to be born (due dates are often miscalculated) and a cervix that isn't ripe. Remember, it's the procedure most likely to lead to a c-section. It's never ideal for a baby to be induced, unless there is a serious, justified, medical reason to do it. Your age is not a medical reason.

# CHAPTER 9

## The Big Event of Birth

### THE POLITICS OF BIRTH – PAST AND PRESENT

The attitudes and practices of childbirth have always reflected society's views on women and sexuality, fulfilling an agenda of some sort. Nothing comparable in a woman's life has been quite so interfered in, disturbed and controlled. The more the *system* got involved in the process, the more the *sacred feminine* was disempowered. Depending on the current belief or latest technology new practices were introduced, without much investigation into the side effects or long-term consequences.

### A GENERAL HISTORY OF BIRTH THROUGH THE AGES[1]

*Primal to Ancient Times*

Women were *givers of life*, connected to Mother Nature and deity. Birth was a celebratory event and linked to cycles (lunar, planting and harvesting). There was widespread belief in ancestral souls and magical powers. It was generally thought that babies started labour and that contractions were just a reaction. Births were generally easy, short and assisted by 'wise women' who used healing herbs and amulets. Upright birth postures were predominant, such as standing, squatting, kneeling and sitting; trees, poles and ropes were used for support. In ancient Egypt women squatted or knelt over birthing bricks, and in Greek and Roman times they often sat on birthing stools. Hippocrates and Aristotle, of the Grecian School of Medicine, never mentioned pain or complicated births in their notes and understood the mind–body connection. They also advocated that there should be no 'meddlesome interference' because 'nature is the best physician'.

## Early Christianity

Icons of female deity were destroyed and old superstitions became Christianized. With the increasing power of the Church, women were pushed into subordinate roles in religion and society. Midwives, healers and wise women became associated with witchcraft as monks and priests took over medical authority. Law decreed that women be segregated during pregnancy and isolated for birth because they were guilty of 'carnal sin'. Midwifery was abolished, leaving labouring women without support; birth became feared as a result. Flawed Bible translations said painful childbirth was punishment for Eve's original sin, otherwise known as 'The Curse of Eve'.

## Mediaeval to Seventeenth Century

Midwifery came back into practice and most births were managed thus. Houses were prepared by closing windows, stopping up keyholes, drawing curtains and lighting candles. The dark, warm atmosphere was supposed to protect from evil spirits and ward off chills. Various birth positions were used but generally it was before the hearth, not in bed. Slow labours were sped by herbs; midwives had methods to turn a badly positioned baby. Male doctors only dealt with emergencies: 'When a man comes, one or both must die.'

## Eighteenth Century

Science became more popular, especially with the upper classes. In the 1740s forceps were popularized but used by many without training. Birth was increasingly seen as dangerous and many women died due to the highly infectious childbirth (puerperal) fever. Around mid-century childbirth customs among the upper classes began to change. Doctors saw the economic advantage of managing birth, and midwives lost respect. Surgeons called for bright, airy rooms rather than dark chambers because they thought it would ward off childbirth fever. In order to justify their presence doctors were more likely to intervene in the birth process with forceps and drugs. Mothers were generally advised to breastfeed and observe a month-long 'lying-in' period. Upper class women hired wet nurses. Lower classes and more traditional families still gave birth the 'old way'.

### TWO FAMOUS MIDWIVES IN HISTORY

*Catherina Schrader*

A Dutch midwife, assisted 3,060 births during her lifetime from 1656 to 1746. She made notes after each delivery. She assisted 70 twin births and two sets of triplets. She performed 88 breech extractions and in six cases of *placenta praevia*, manual removal of the placenta and extraction of the baby. Her overall maternal mortality rate was 5 per cent, which is less than the figure reached in the US in 1936.

> *Martha Ballard*
> Assisted nearly 1,000 births in Maine, US during her life and
> recorded 814 deliveries between 1785 and 1812 in her diary.
> Martha waded through hip-deep snowdrifts and crossed
> frozen rivers to get to labouring mothers. She lost only five
> mothers, none during delivery. She was a healer, with a good
> understanding of medicinal herbs.

## Nineteenth Century

The campaign against the 'uneducated' midwives continued as
women were pushed out of 'rational science' in order to assume a
strictly domestic role. The superiority of the male surgeon at delivery
was accepted everywhere in Europe and middle-class America.
Puerperal fever reached catastrophic proportions (for example,
the maternal mortality rose to 49 per cent in Vienna's university
clinic in the 1840s). It was discovered in the late 1840s that the
disease was spread by surgeons performing vaginal examinations
with unclean hands ('the physician and the disease entered hand
in hand into the chamber of the unsuspecting patient'). By the
middle of the century (Victorian era) there was an increasing view
that civilized ladies were too fragile to give birth as the 'savages'
did. Due to corseting, overindulgence and inactivity, women were
unhealthier. They delivered lying down, anaesthetized and with the
aid of instruments such as forceps. Pain-relief became fashionable
and sought after by mothers, particularly chloroform and ether;
this resulted in many children being born sick, and mothers who
overdosed during childbirth. It also started the trend of giving birth
in hospital, where it was possible to administer anaesthesia. *Pap,* a
mix of bread, water and sugar, was fed to newborns. Old rituals of
childbirth continued in poor, rural areas, but even here they started
to dwindle. The caesarean section was performed successfully in
1882 thanks to new antiseptic measures.

## Twentieth Century

In 1900, the majority of deliveries still occurred at home; male physicians attended nearly all births and midwives took care of those who couldn't afford a doctor. By the 1920s doctors believed that 'normal' deliveries were so rare that 'routine interventions' (including sedation, episiotomy and forceps delivery) were performed during labour to prevent trouble. Despite the trend for more doctor-led hospital births, maternal mortality peaked between 1900 and 1930, with 600 to 700 deaths per 100,000 births. The number of infant deaths also increased partly due to excessive or improperly performed intervention. In 1914, doctors in Germany started using *Daemmerschlaf* or *Twilight Sleep*, and the trend rapidly spread. Originally welcomed as a way of managing pain, it took decades to see how brutal this mixture of morphine and scopolamine was. It only numbed pain marginally and induced a state of disorientation, meaning mothers had no memory of the birth process. The narcotics drove many into a hallucinatory frenzy; they would thrash wildly and bang their heads so that they were shackled or tied down, and padded to avoid strap-marks and bruises. Some had their legs clamped in stirrups for hours until the doctors arrived and pulled drugged babies out of the birth canal with instruments. Twilight sleep became the most popular form of managing childbirth in the 1930s and 1940s, and didn't go out of fashion in the US until the 1960s or even 1970s.

The British doctor Grantly Dick-Read published *Birth without Fear* in 1933, based on his experiences watching women give birth painlessly in London's East End slums and First World War trenches. He said fear and tension were to blame for suffering and that women could be educated to make childbirth a joyous experience. But his ideas were marginalized by the medical establishment. By 1960 practically all births took place in hospital under continuous foetal monitoring. Mothers were routinely separated from newborns, who slept in nurseries and were fed formula milk.

In 1974 Frederick Leboyer published *Birth without Violence*. Explaining birth from the baby's point of view, he advocated a fearless, trauma-free transition from womb to world. Another Frenchman, Michel Odent, introduced the concepts of birthing pools and home-like birthing rooms. In the US, Ina May Gaskin set up The Farm Midwifery Center, giving direct-entry midwifery a boost. Based on the midwives' good birth outcomes, with impressively low rates of medical intervention, she published *Spiritual Midwifery* in 1975. Consumer groups and women's movements began criticizing the aggressive management of childbirth in hospitals, and the natural birth movement gained momentum. However, the medical establishment discouraged home births, claiming them to be dangerous; in some places in the US they were even made illegal. Epidural anaesthesia started becoming available in hospitals by the mid-1970s, giving women a further option for 'pain-free' childbirth.

## Our Industrialized, Electronic Age

Most births today occur in a highly medicalized, techno-centric environment. Big factors at play are time and money. Hospital institutions have protocols to fulfil and rigid safety precautions to follow. A system that focuses on managing risk can lead to unnecessary procedures. It's the priority of obstetrics to control childbirth. Artificial inducement, labour augmentation and intervention are still standard birth procedures and routinely administered without any justification. Hospital staff rely on expensive gadgetry and drugs because it's the only model they were trained in. Added to this there is an increasing fear of litigation which fuels the urge to rush and control birth as much as possible. Caesareans are regularly performed because they're doctor-friendly, over in 20 minutes, less likely to lead to lawsuits and – here comes the really cynical bit – they bring in a lot more cash.

**BIRTH ON TIME**

According to statistics, most births take place from Monday to Friday between 9 a.m. and 5 p.m. There is a surge in births just before the Christmas holidays begin. Now doesn't that make you wonder?

## Safe Birth

If you're constantly told that *something could go wrong*, you start believing it. In most people's minds birth is an urgent medical process, because that is the way we've seen it in films and on television. There is a tendency to dramatize birth risks, despite the fact that perinatal and maternal mortality are at all-time lows. Thanks to improved health, cleanliness and methods to treat existing pathologies, giving birth has never been so safe. It's NOT the shift to hospital births and increased intervention that has improved the perinatal mortality rate; the advent of antibiotics, blood-banking and healthier mothers are the reasons birth has become safer.[2] So maybe we need to trust the genuinely scientific evidence?

We have enough clear data to seriously question the industrialized, obstetric approach to childbirth. Evidence from official statistics and specific studies consistently finds that a non-medical environment leads to lower rates of infant mortality, maternal mortality and fewer caesarean sections.

## How Normal Is a Natural, Complication-free Birth?

- When The Farm Midwifery Center was founded in the early 1970s, 186 women gave birth without any surgical or medical intervention; for birth 187, the first c-section proved necessary. The second c-section wasn't needed until birth number 324. Four decades and thousands of births later, the c-section rate at The Farm is still below 2 per cent (in many US hospitals it stands between 40 and 50 per cent), fewer than 1 per cent of births involve forceps or vacuum extractors, and none is drug-assisted, except in a few cases of medical emergencies. Over 95 per cent are home births.

- In 1753 the encyclopaedist William Smellie estimated that 92 per cent of births could be natural.
- Natural, spontaneous childbirth occurred in 94 per cent of Catherina Schrader's practice (see page 193).
- World Health Organization statistics show that 85–90 per cent of women will have a problem-free labour.
- The HypnoBirthing pioneer Marie Mongan believes 95 per cent of women can give birth comfortably.
- Two large studies following healthy women who gave birth outside hospital with a trained midwife showed that 95 per cent had normal, vaginal deliveries and healthy babies.

The National Patient Safety Agency examined 60,000 maternity ward errors between November 2003 and June 2006 and found that nearly 18,000 labouring women had been injured unnecessarily; 1,000 of these injuries were serious. The NHS gets 10 complaints a day about birth experiences.

## A Comparison

### Netherlands

Holland has the highest national rate of home births in the industrialized world (30 per cent) and a notably low caesarean rate (between 2 and 6 per cent). Home births in Holland have a perinatal mortality rate (including transfers) seven times lower than the perinatal mortality in hospitals. If a Dutch woman says she's going to hospital to give birth, everyone will ask, 'Why, what's wrong?' Independent midwives handle 75 per cent of all births. Are Dutch women more birth-talented? No, it is simply that the inquisition against midwives didn't happen in the Netherlands.

## United States

The US has the world's most expensive maternity care but one of the highest infant mortality rates in the Western world, behind 40 other nations. The maternal mortality rate is more than twice that of Holland. The caesarean rate increased by 50 per cent from 1996 to 2006 and it currently stands at 31 per cent; higher than most industrialized countries. Only 0.5 per cent of births take place at home. Due to the country's private medical and insurance system, doctors make more money if they perform more procedures. In this fiercely competitive market, midwives have been driven underground by obstetricians who control 92 per cent of all births. Due to strong lobbying by doctors, The American Medical Association claims home birth is dangerous, thus most insurance companies won't cover it. Amnesty International has dubbed the US record on childbirth a 'human rights crisis' due to systematic failures and violation of women's rights.

> *'We have destroyed obstetrics; the profession has downgraded its skills and knowledge has deteriorated. Doctors don't know physiological birth any more, they just learn about surgery. Birth outcomes are worse than ever. The US model is now even reaching countries in the East like India.'*

INA MAY GASKIN, AUTHOR AND FOUNDER OF
THE FARM MIDWIFERY CENTER

# FROM FEAR AND PAIN TO BLISS

*Myths and Fear*

We sadly lost a lot of the knowledge about pain-free childbirth in our society over the centuries. The thinking that childbirth is dangerous and painful is still reflected in our current birth practices. Cultural conditioning has led us to fear this primal act that connects us with our true power. Countless women before us have indeed endured torturous and deadly birth experiences, often due to inadequate hygiene or the heavy-handed medical intervention that was intended to help them. Modern technology is very good at saving lives, but we should realize that in a birthing situation it's the technology that usually causes the problem in the first place.

With today's knowledge and the extraordinary health we enjoy compared to our predecessors, there's no reason to fear childbirth. We are safe wherever we give birth and can rely on emergency facilities as back-up. To embrace birth as the truly amazing experience it is, we need to let go of fear. Fear is very contagious. It enslaves us and creates a submissive victim consciousness. Why should we hand over this most important, life-affirming event? Ladies! It's time to take our power, dignity and freedom back.

*'What I'd say to women is get out of that medicalized system. Our psyche is so caught up in what the medical system says we don't even own our own bodies.'*
DR CHRISTIANE NORTHRUP

## Perfect Design

The female body is designed perfectly for birth. The uterus is actually a muscle that begins gently pushing the baby down once labour has begun. One could say that labour is simply the opening of a very strong muscle. The cervix, which is closed in pregnancy to keep the baby in, also consists of muscular tissues and gradually opens during labour. The ligaments that join the four bones of the pelvis soften during pregnancy to prepare for delivery. This means that even the biggest baby can pass without injury. Meanwhile the brain produces powerful endorphins during labour. These neuropeptides are hundreds of times more powerful than morphine and a far better analgesic painkiller than any drug. They have such a tranquillizing effect that a woman can cut herself off from the world and go deep into a place where the process of birth unfolds instinctively. I first observed this when I attended a friend's birth. There was a moment when her eyes glazed over and she went to *that place of less pain.* The transition was a miracle to watch and a smooth delivery of her son followed soon after. A birth like this can have a profound effect upon your life because it puts you in touch with the immense inner resources you're capable of.

## Managing Pain

If we approach labour being afraid, stress hormones are released and there is a kind of *freeze* effect as the arteries going to the uterus tense up. The blood and oxygen supply is restricted further, tensing up the muscles in the uterus and the cervix. If muscles work against each other, it's painful. And if the baby's head is pushed against firmly closed lower muscles that won't relax, it can result in a drawn-out, painful labour.

If you think you have unresolved or psychological fears to do with birth, it's worth preparing well, through rebirthing or hypnotherapy, for example. Remember the mind–body connection: the mind believes and the body follows. In ancient times we used birthing rituals and called upon spiritual and protective powers to guide us. Modern medicine has replaced rituals and dehumanized the process. This is why it's important to surround yourself with positive birth stories and images. We have rituals for other milestones of our lives, so why not create your own for this key experience?

Upright postures were used in ancient times and they are still used by ethnic groups around the world. Standing, sitting or crouching can help dilation and make it easier for the baby's head to emerge. Also, rather than fighting labour, tensing up and screaming 'No' (which causes the body to contract), embrace the contractions or surges with a 'Yes' to open (you don't have to physically say *yes*; thinking it is enough). Circling or spiralling your hips is also known to help as this is the basic movement of energy that can be found everywhere in the universe, from strands of DNA to the shape of galaxies.

Ina May Gaskin talks about labouring women being elemental forces like a tidal wave, tornado or volcano. Birth is about *going into*, rather than *against* this primal energy.

Another skewed concept is forced pushing. It's counter-productive because it can close the lower vaginal muscles, create stress and slow down the actual birth. Women who are drugged can't feel the contractions, which is why they're told to push. But when childbirth is controlled by the labouring woman, her body opens naturally rather than being coached by well-meaning attendants shouting 'Push!' HypnoBirthers talk about *breathing the baby down*, and Dr Michel Odent speaks of the *foetus ejection reflex*, which is triggered by a rush of adrenalin.

> **'Mental fear leads to physical tension leads to needless pain,' was Grantly Dick-Read's conclusion in the 1930s. As the woman in the East End slums said to him after birthing her baby without any help or fuss; 'It didn't hurt. It wasn't supposed to, was it, Doctor?'**

## Beating the 'It's So Painful' Hysteria

Why do mothers tell other women – the ones who are pregnant or haven't given birth yet – their horror stories concerning birth? Is it some kind of macho, *look at my scars* competition, so typical of our culture? Putting fear in a mother-to-be is unsupportive and misleading. Every woman should be given the chance to approach her birth with hope, courage and optimism. Birth is one of the most important, intense and potentially beautiful experiences of your life; so don't let anyone spoil it for you. If you're a woman with a bad birth story – KEEP IT TO YOURSELF – until after the woman you want to share your story with can share hers, too.

## In Touch with Instinct

The ideal conditions of birth are quite simple, as Michel Odent says: 'One cannot help a physiological process. The point is not to hinder it.'

According to Dr Odent and other childbirth experts, a woman in labour needs privacy and security in order to reduce the activity of the neocortex. This 'rational brain' or 'brain of the intellect' is specifically human and it inhibits the birth process. If the labouring woman can reduce the activity of the human brain and let the mammalian, instinctive brain take over, she'll be able to go to 'another world'. Then the hormones necessary will be excreted and she gives birth more easily. That is why a woman in labour needs to be protected from any sort of stimulation of the intellectual brain, such as language or too many people around. She shouldn't be disturbed, interrupted or distracted. Nor should the labour process be interfered with because it could upset the birthing hormones and delicate balance. These basic needs for privacy and security are ones all other mammals will seek out when giving birth; they'll usually hide and isolate themselves. Any signs of danger or attempts to move them to a new environment will disturb labour; in some cases it will even stop. Mice giving birth in glass cages will have more problems than those who are hidden from view. Birthing women in more primitive societies are thought to give birth easily because they do it in complete privacy.

> *'The vagina does not open well when there are people in the room harassing and frightening the mother. The mind controls the body; any kind of threat and the blood won't flow to that part of the body. A man won't get an erection with people watching and telling him to hurry up. For so long we have dismissed the whole idea that mother's feelings don't matter. Of course they do.'*
>
> INA MAY GASKIN

Avoid if you can multiple vaginal exams, continuous foetal monitoring, artificial rupture of membranes and birth-induction drugs.

## Indigenous Birth

> *'The cultures having the greatest respect for life, for Mother Earth – such as the Maoris, the Pygmies, the Huichols – are also those that disturb the mother–baby relationship as little as possible.'[3]*
>
> MICHEL ODENT

The Pygmies are an interesting example because they have very brief and easy births, despite the fact that Pygmy babies are proportionally the biggest in the world – about one-tenth of their mother's body weight (which would be like us giving birth to 14-pound babies). When labour commences the Pygmy mother walks to the river with two midwives, singing and being joyful. The mother and the midwives breathe deeply together when the time comes, experiencing a 'tremendous feeling of oneness'. The mother will sing another song after the birth of her child to celebrate. When she returns to the village the father greets the child and thanks his wife.[4]

## Gentle Birth Options for You and the Baby

*Hypnotherapy* – Studies have shown hypnotherapy to be more effective than some of the strongest painkillers. Through self-hypnosis, positive thinking, breathing and visualization, deep levels of relaxation can be reached. To understand the technique consult tutors, books or videos.

*Active Birthing* – An approach that emphasizes empowerment and natural birth physiology. You can do a course during pregnancy (some evenings or a two-day intensive) where you will learn breathing, relaxation and instinctual movements in supported upright positions. This includes massage and positive visualizations for labour and birth, and is very inclusive of partners.

*The Gentle Birth Method* – 'The Jeyarani Way' offers a birth-preparation programme to pregnant mothers that includes Josephson's creative healing massage technique, reflexology, Ayurveda, Bowen therapy, cranio-sacral therapy and weekly self-hypnosis birth-preparation classes all the way through pregnancy.

*Calm Birth* – This uses meditation and the latest findings in mind/body medicine for an easy, empowering birth.

*Relaxed breathing* – Yoga, meditation and breathing techniques can be used to ride the surges of labour and relax into childbirth.

*Acupuncture and acupressure* – Studies have shown that needles or pressure in certain locations trigger the release of endorphins which block pain signals. It has been widely used in the East during childbirth for centuries. Stimulating the flow of Qi energy is believed to release the blockages that cause pain.

*Reflexology* – By massaging certain areas of the feet the uterus can be relaxed and the pituitary gland stimulated to reduce pain and shorten labour. Studies show that reflexology also leads to fewer caesarean interventions.

*Massage* – Your partner, a doula or therapist massages sore spots to ease pain.

*Hydrotherapy* – Warm water relaxes tense muscles and eases pains. You may even want to deliver in the tub.

*Aromatherapy* – Essential oils combined with massage can relieve back pain and increase relaxation.

*Bach Flower remedies* – The remedies can relax you and make you feel better. Ideally used combined with other therapies such as reflexology.

*Homeopathy* – Ask the homeopath to give you a remedy for anxiety, exhaustion or pain.


## *The Biochemical Perfection of Love, Labour and Birth*

Since science discovered how neurotransmitters work, it's clear that childbirth can be a sensual, sexual experience. The love hormone, oxytocin, which causes contractions during labour, is also present in lovemaking (having a baby really has a lot in common with making one). During labour the brain increases the release of powerful beta-endorphins: natural opiates of pleasure. These are responsible for numbing pain and taking you to a euphoric, altered state of consciousness; i.e. from pain to pleasure. Once you've reached this blissful, ecstatic, even spiritual state there is a rush of adrenalin shortly before birth. This intense moment helps birth the baby and is neurologically and physically very similar to orgasm. The highest levels of oxytocin a woman will ever have are in the moments after she has given birth to a baby. One could say that this is the closest to 'God' or 'Pure Love' a woman can come. The hormones are in an elevated ecstatic state for about an hour, as if nature has perfectly arranged it for mother and child to find that moment of connection and intimacy in order to fall in love.

A biological imprint is created in the bonding circuits between the two.

## How Was It for the Baby?

Birth is a key moment for human beings. It brings an end to the secure time we spent in the womb and is a crucial moment for the development of our adaptive systems. The period that follows birth will never happen again with such intensity; and it literally affects our capacity to love. Microbiologists and researchers from the fast-evolving field of primal health say that we remember the womb and being born in every cell of our body. Birth memory can affect your entire life and personality, even though there will be no conscious memory of it. Due to limbic imprinting, birth and early childhood are our comfort zones, so we recreate these experiences, conditions and feelings subconsciously throughout life.

## Epidural

If you've read all the above and you still think, 'No way, I'm not doing even a little bit of pain' there is a more radical form of pain-relief available. You can have an epidural as soon as the first contraction sets in. Alternatively you might feel you need one if labour goes on for too long or does end up becoming more painful than you'd hoped. It's not a crime. You won't be ostracized by the 'no-drugs girls', nor will they get badges or be better mothers. Many women have given birth easily and comfortably with epidurals.

The advantages are that you are only anaesthetized from the waist downwards, so you are still conscious to witness the birth. There are, however, some disadvantages:

1.  You won't have the oxytocin rush just mentioned.
2.  A huge, hollow needle will be stuck into your spine (and you thought childbirth hurt!).

3. You can't get in the birthing pool and you'll be attached to an IV.
4. Your blood pressure can drop and there are some rare cases of blood-clotting complications.
5. If spinal fluid leaks you can end up with severe headaches for hours or even days.
6. Labour can slow down.
7. Your baby can get distressed (that's why its heartbeat will be continuously monitored).
8. There is an increased likelihood of ending up with a forceps, suction or caesarean delivery.

> **'Take anything they'll give you. Childbirth is not the time to say no to drugs.'**
>
> ADVICE GIVEN TO ME IN A LADIES' LOO WHEN I WAS
> 8 MONTHS PREGNANT

Other forms of pain-relief are Entonox (gas and air) and pethidine. Entonox works for some women, but others find it makes them feel sick and dries out the mouth. Pethidine is an analgesic often used to dull pain and relax the mother. It can make you very drowsy and even sick and it crosses into the placenta to the baby with the same effects, often making the baby too tired to drink when it's born. General anaesthesia is rarely used because it knocks out the baby as well as the mother and can leave children with motor-skill difficulties and disturbed behaviour that linger long after birth.

## ALL THOSE BIRTH OPTIONS

Admittedly it is overwhelming. The internet is saturated with information, each person you know will recommend another approach and your own mother is likely to have a fit if you suggest you're considering a home or water birth.

## Home Birth

There's an increasing trend to give birth at home, which is, theoretically, encouraged by the NHS. Home is the environment that is most conducive to the birthing process because it's familiar and provides the most privacy and least interference. It also means you don't have to travel anywhere during contractions. Bonding with a newborn baby is easier at home than anywhere else.

To be able to use an NHS midwife, you have to be considered low-risk. Unless you have any other known complications, a first-time birth at an increased age *is* in the low-risk bracket, despite what anyone might try to tell you (the in-laws usually have very strong opinions on this one). Mention to sceptics the example of Holland; you can also find home birth stories to inspire you on the internet (www.homebirth.org.uk). If you feel confident enough that a home birth is want you want, insist on staying put.

> 'I'm really indecisive, anxious and cautious normally. I'm nervous about lots of things like driving a car. But in birth it's like a primeval me took over and made decisions. I have never felt stronger or more capable.'
>
> MARGARET, HOME BIRTH AT 38

It's been proven that home births are at least as safe[5] if not safer than birthing in a hospital or clinic.[6] With many wards dirty, and antibiotic-resistant hospital bugs on the increase, home is the better place for mother and newborn in terms of infections. Remember that if things don't go according to plan, the midwives will arrange a hospital transfer ahead of time; they don't wait for a real emergency to present itself. Midwives also have emergency drugs for post-partum haemorrhage and basic medical equipment including infant resuscitators. The first steps taken in these very rare cases are the same as in hospital anyway. A study showed it took on average 43 minutes for the surgical team to perform an in-labour 'emergency' caesarean due to foetal distress,[7] so this means that a patient already in hospital isn't on the operating table any faster than someone transferring from home (providing you don't live at the end of Loch Ness, of course!).

> *'I was 42 when I had my fourth child. I'd previously had surgery on my uterus and if I'd have gone to hospital they'd have treated me as a high-risk case. But I wanted a normal and natural birth if possible. I stayed at home and felt confident. I knew the hospital was 5 minutes away, I had nothing to be afraid of. My body knew what to do. The birth was intense and efficient. My son was born while I was standing up – and he was a 5-kilo baby. Anyone that age wanting to give birth at home would be wise to search out those who have knowledge and trust in the birth process, and choose them as birth attendants.'*
>
> JANET BALASKAS, ACTIVE BIRTH FOUNDER

Some birthing women like to have various birth attendants, such as a good friend, doula or family members around. Various experts in the field of birthing discourage having too many people around (especially if it's your first birth) because it can interfere in the labour process and make it more stressful for you. So pick your inner circle carefully; anyone who hasn't healed their own birth trauma is likely to project this fear onto you. Ideally your attendants will be helpful when needed but discreetly stay in the background and be able to handle the intensity of the energy.

When it comes to husbands, this can also be quite contentious. A dominant husband who acts like a coach is no good, neither is a nervous partner with birth fears. Even though it's not politically correct to say, women tend to do better in birth when husbands leave. In societies where mothers give birth easily, birth is considered a woman's business. If men play a role, it's supportive on the periphery, fetching things and making the woman feel protected and safe.

Michel Odent suggests having nobody around during labour, apart from an experienced, motherly midwife with a low level of adrenalin – an image he often uses is that of a *knitting midwife*.

> **'If you can choose a midwife, choose one who has the highest capacity to keep her mouth closed.'**
> MICHEL ODENT

If your baby is in a more difficult position for birth or you want to have a VBAC (Vaginal Birth after Caesarean), look for a midwife with experience in this area. In some cases the NHS may not provide one but you always have the option of using an independent midwife; you would, however, have to cover the cost yourself.

## Water Birth

Water has a very relaxing and softening effect on a labouring woman's muscles and her perineum. It is also shown to increase the production of oxytocin and endorphins. Entering a birthing pool at the right time – when you are about 5 cm dilated – can help labour to progress; an added bonus is that it provides you with privacy. The foetus has spent 9 months swimming in amniotic fluid, so being born into water is a gentle way to transition from womb to world. However, many women will come out of the birthing pool in the last minute because they feel more comfortable delivering on 'dry land'. Water has healing qualities and has been used for birth since ancient times. The Maoris frequently birthed in tidepools near the ocean, and in Polynesia they used the warm lagoons created by coral reefs. There was also a *conscious birth* movement in the 1980s near Odessa in Russia, where babies were regularly born into the Black Sea. These days you can hire or buy a birthing pool for home use; many birthing centres in the UK also have pools.

## Birthing Centre

Some women want the option of a natural birth but feel more confident near hospital facilities. Birthing centres are now mostly midwife-led, and this tends to lead to fewer interventions. Many centres in the UK today are well equipped with more homely-looking birthing rooms and birthing pools. They can administer oxygen and IVs but most are affiliated to hospitals, for easy transfer if complications arise or you want an epidural. The main disadvantage is that facilities, staff and attitudes towards birth differ from place to place, so research well beforehand. Many places are understaffed and will want you to birth as efficiently as possible.

'Failure to progress' often leads to a hospital transfer, even if that's not what you had planned. Centres have to fulfil certain protocols and these systems are hard to shake, especially if you're a novice in the area of birth. It's not easy arguing with a bossy midwife when you're in labour. Decisions are made quickly and your time in the birthing room is limited because you're 'occupying valuable space'. Don't make the mistake of checking in too early; arriving in an advanced phase of labour means you'll be more likely to stay put until after birth.

> 'When I went into the clinic the first thing they tried to do was stick an IV in my arm. I literally had to push the midwife away. If it weren't for my birth attendant Pat they would have got their way and given me all the drugs. I would really recommend taking a good female friend or someone in with you to do all the negotiating. It's almost like you need a lawyer there to keep those people at bay.'
>
> **CARLA, BABIES AT 40 AND 42**

## I'M OLDER, WHAT'S DIFFERENT?

If you're healthy and fit, there's no reason why birth should be any more difficult than for a younger woman. It's usually other people's attitudes, rather than your age, that's the problem. Older first-time mothers may be more afraid and take an approach that is rather 'cerebral'. The attitudes of the caregivers will also influence levels of anxiety and choices made. Because fast childbirth is the goal today, when labour takes over 24 hours people start worrying about potential risks and dangers to the baby. Studies show that the high levels of obstetric intervention (inductions, augmentation of labour, assisted deliveries and caesareans) experienced by older first-time mothers are not explained by actual complications.[8] This means that in the great majority of cases intervention is not medically justified. So all those finger-pointers who say older mothers are a drain on the NHS should question the systems in place instead.

*'Birth isn't harder when you're older. Whoever arbitrarily decided this didn't have a good reason. I've seen many amazing births to women over 40. If it's a first-time birth there may be more fears to overcome and it may take longer if the woman hasn't prepared well. But there is a great range that is still within normal.'*

INA MAY GASKIN

*'In my experience older pregnant women are more body aware than younger women who are more distracted. They do very well at birth because they listen to the instructions on breathing and do it right.'*

FRANÇOISE BARBIRA FREEDMAN, PREGNANCY YOGA PIONEER AND

BIRTHLIGHT FOUNDER

*'When there are no tangible medical complications of pregnancy, the risks of childbirth in older women are no greater than in younger women.'*

BRITISH JOURNAL OF OBSTETRICS AND GYNAECOLOGY[9]

> Choosing the right birth environment and the right caregivers is probably the most important decision you can make for your birth, because it influences the outcome.

## Midwives

There are big differences in attitude and experience: some midwives are very technology-focused, others support a completely drug-free home birth, and others are in the middle. It's a good idea to ask what their birth philosophy is beforehand.

## Birthing Centre, Clinic or Hospital

Make sure staff support your wishes during birth and that they leave your baby with you after it's born.

Ideally the following would apply:

- Induction rate of less than 10 per cent
- Episiotomy rate of less than 10 per cent
- Caesarean rate of less than 10 per cent (less than 15 per cent in hospitals treating high-risk cases)
- No routine practices such as IVs, membrane rupturing, electronic foetal monitoring or labour augmentation through synthetic oxytocin.

*'I was a midwife for 12 years but stopped because I couldn't bear the way women were being treated any more. Hospital policies are not for the benefit*

*of women, nor are they consistent or designed on evidence-based practice. Policy differs from one hospital to another and it doesn't relate to any research – it's basically made up. I saw many women who had unnecessary caesareans and were pressured or bullied because they couldn't make decisions. A lot of women are assaulted during birth and traumatized. I found my own births totally pain-free and sincerely believe we are so conditioned to expect pain that we create it.'*

FIONA, EX-MIDWIFE AND HYPNOBIRTHING TUTOR

## Hospital

For any medical procedures such as an epidural or caesarean you'll have to go to hospital. Once there, you're basically a patient and will generally be told what to do. If this is what you want, then just lie back and enjoy the high-tech ride. With the right attitude there's no reason why hospital can't be a good – and even empowering – experience. I know plenty of women where it worked out well with helpful, competent staff looking after them. Your baby can still come into the world gently, despite the clinical circumstances; you might just have to work a little harder at insisting on things being done a certain way.

'Behind the successful and blissful birth of my identical twins by caesarean there was a solid foundation of bureaucratic manoeuvring, successfully negotiated by an amazing community midwife. Once researched and written, the birth plan, like a contract between lawyers, went backwards and forwards by email between community midwife, consultant, theatre director, doula and me until the "agreement" was honed, refined and signed off. It took months, but was essential for the happy outcome. One area of discussion was my wish to have skin-to-skin with the babies straight away in theatre. In most cases it is not possible because the theatre is kept at a very cool temperature. The compromise was to have the babies wrapped up with staff in the theatre helping me to feed them straight away. Love poured out everywhere and both the doula and the wonderful community midwife said they had never seen twins simultaneously breastfeeding in theatre before. It was the most ideal caesarean I could have had.'

CAMILLA, TWINS AT 43

## What the Baby Likes

- Dimmed lights and a warm room
- Having the umbilical cord cut only once it has stopped pulsating
- Being placed on its mother skin-to-skin immediately after birth, and staying there
- Eye-to-eye contact with mother (and father)
- No unnecessary checks, eye drops, shots or vaccines (vitamin K is unnecessary whether you're breastfeeding or bottle feeding; Hepatitis B is a sexually transmitted disease, the vaccine does more harm than good at this stage)
- Any physical assessment by the nurse should be done while the baby is on its mother. If the baby needs to be taken away, ideally the father will carry it
- No rubbing or washing of its sensitive skin to clean the vernix
- Weighing, measuring or any necessary tests only after the initial feeding
- Being in mother's arms as much as possible (after 9 months inside, this is the next 'womb space')
- Having enough room and allowing for colostrum feeds as often as needed (colostrum is the first milk you'll produce; it contains vital antibodies and is higher in fat and protein). Most hospital beds are too narrow to accommodate having the baby in bed but bassinets are provided.

- Lots of cuddles, kisses and sounds it recognizes, such as mum and dad's voices
- Being around the smells it recognizes (mum and dad).

## Immediate Aftermath

It's important there are no distractions after the baby's born in order for you to birth the placenta. Delaying clamping the umbilical cord will help delivery, as will squatting or kneeling. Too many people fussing may get in the way of you bonding with your baby and the love hormone, oxytocin, doing its job. If you avoid bathing the baby for the first day its incredible scent will activate your mothering instinct and lactating hormones. If you intend to breastfeed, make it clear you don't want the baby to be fed any formula milk because your milk production won't be stimulated the way it should be. The early colostrum feeds, until your milk comes in, are most important. Breastfeeding will also help your uterus to contract, shrink and stop bleeding. Research shows that breastfeeding within the first hour improves infant survival and increases the duration of exclusive nursing.

> *'The best way to sabotage breastfeeding is to take the baby away from the mother [during] those crucial hours after birth.'*
>
> INA MAY GASKIN

# CAESAREANS AND OTHER INTERVENTIONS

## Induction and Labour Augmentation

The most common birth intervention is induction or labour augmentation through synthetic oxytocin. In most countries synthetic oxytocin does not appear in the birth statistics, probably because it isn't administered by a doctor. Most frequently used are syntocinon, prostaglandin E, pitocin and misoprostol. A big problem with all these drugs is that they make your contractions much stronger and unnaturally painful; so painful that many women ask for an epidural. You won't be free to move around to 'take the pain' because you'll be attached to a drip as well as to monitoring equipment. Babies often get distressed when these drugs are introduced to the birthing process, and so the likelihood of ending up with a surgical birth shoots up. If it's your first baby, induction doubles your chances of having a caesarean. Another disadvantage is that synthetic oxytocin blocks the release of natural oxytocin, so your brain will not be able to release the incredible maternal love hormones during and after birth.

A study of 120 new mothers in a London hospital found that 40 per cent considered their first emotional reaction to holding their child after birth to be indifference.[10]

Women over 35 are more likely to be coerced into induction and labour augmentation. But please remember that age is *not* a reason to interfere in your birthing process. If you're not feeling stressed by the situation, then you should be allowed to birth in your own time.

'They gave me prostaglandin to increase the contractions but the pain then became too much. It was like I was in drug rehab: I was sweating, vomiting and had diarrhoea. I kept trying to breathe like I'd learned in yoga, but the drugs were too strong. Eventually I asked for an epidural but then labour stopped, the monitor showed the baby was distressed and I ended up with a caesarean.'
ANNE-MARIE, BABIES AT 36 AND 40

## The Effects of Childbirth Drugs on Babies

Whether it's for pain-relief or induction, drugs desensitize the oxytocin receptors of mother and child, inhibiting bonding and breastfeeding. Because medical research is very expensive and time-consuming, most drugs will be implemented if no serious adverse effects for the mother or baby are immediately found, even if the long-term effects have not been officially established. 'Safe until proven dangerous' is the general attitude in obstetrics to drugs – this from a profession that does not have such a good history of practice when it comes to drugs.

Drugs that are new to induction such as misoprostol (Cytotec) are regularly given without informed consent. Its use is controversial and has been associated with serious complications including uterine rupture. Various independent studies have found that using drugs during childbirth can have negative long-term consequences for the child such as drug addiction and autism.[11] Studies also showed that traumatic birth experiences increase the risk of adolescent violent behaviour and suicide.[12]

## ELECTRONIC FOETAL MONITORING

Overwhelming scientific evidence has shown that electronic foetal monitoring does not improve the pregnancy outcome or prevent neonatal death. The only effect monitoring has is increasing the rate of caesareans and forceps deliveries because it creates so many false alarms.[13] Also intermittent monitoring has been proven to be just as effective as continuous monitoring. The costs for the health services are huge. The US, for example, spends about $400 million a year on foetal monitoring alone.

## Episiotomy

What used to be a 'routine cut' is happily making its way into the history books of obstetrics. Studies have shown that this perineum cut can lead to more infections and serious tearing, so that mothers are better off without it. Doctors today should only perform an episiotomy for very good reasons.

## Forceps

These cold, surgical tongs are also making their way into the history books, and many practitioners are reluctant – or have not even been trained – to use them. Forceps are considered in only a small percentage of cases, for example to rotate the baby's head if it's in an unfavourable position. The cervix will have to be fully dilated and an episiotomy is made. There can be some swelling on the baby's scalp, which usually goes away after a few days. These days c-sections are preferred because it is allegedly less traumatic for the baby and the mother.

## Vacuum Extraction

The extractor or ventouse is a plastic cup that sucks the baby out of the birth canal by its head. It does the same job as forceps but is generally implemented more often because it's easier on the vagina. Around 5 per cent of deliveries happen this way.

## Caesareans

Caesarean sections are without a doubt one of the main advances in the field of childbirth. They're fantastic operations which – used for the right reasons – can genuinely save you and your child from a life-threatening situation. But unfortunately today they're used far too often. England's c-section rate is 24.6 per cent, a figure considerably higher than the 10–15 per cent the World Health Organization recommends for industrialized nations. A caesarean costs four times more than a vaginal birth. It would cause serious debt problems for an NHS hospital to reduce its c-section rate. Talk about mixed-up priorities.

Many women now 'elect' to have caesareans for various reasons: the doctor may recommend it, they're afraid of pain or want to schedule a birth into their itinerary. This is of course a personal choice, but avoid it if you can. Unless it's medically justified, it's not in the baby's interest to be 'born' before it's ready. You also mustn't forget that this is major abdominal surgery which will take much longer to recover from. Layers of skin, nerves and meridians are severed. There's also a higher risk for the mother of infection, neural damage and even death: 400 times more women die from c-sections than vaginal births. Babies born this way have more respiratory problems and can be less 'robust' because they're deprived of the beneficial bacteria they're supposed to pick up in the birth canal. The sensory nervous system is also 'switched on' by vaginal birth.

Caesareans are statistically more common amongst later mothers. The reasons are mixed and have to do with personal choices, the attitude of caregivers, the birthing environment and often a lack of options. However, according to my survey, 24 per cent of women over 35 had a caesarean – this included in-labour and elective – so that is within the national norm.

## ACCEPTING THE BIRTH YOU'VE HAD

Birth is one of the most spontaneous events in our lives, where it's best not to get 'stuck in your own script'. Hopefully everything ended happily and you have a healthy baby, even if birth didn't go the way you'd have liked. Even if those first moments weren't ideal, oxytocin will continue to pulse to make your baby feel safe, secure and loved. If, further along the line, you think your child is crying needlessly, look into cranio-sacral osteopathy – this can work wonders for infants with birth trauma. Women often feel angry, sad, cheated or even depressed after a negative birth experience but there are many ways to find healing. The best thing you can take away is the knowledge of how to approach it next time. You didn't fail; you did the best you could under the circumstances.

Don't stop believing in your ability or the perfect design of your body. Justifications like 'The baby's head was too big and your pelvis was too narrow' or 'The baby's head was stuck, you both could have died,' are misinformed judgements just fuelling the negative myths. Every birth is different, and just because this one was difficult doesn't mean future ones will be. Many women go on to have easy, pain-free, uncomplicated births after an ordeal the first time round, and 70 per cent of mothers who had caesareans go on to have a vaginal birth.

NB: Do read the first short sections of Chapters 10 and 11 soon, which are all about the immediate aftermath (what on earth to do with the baby all day long once you get home) and the all-important post-birth recovery period.

## Fearless Future

From statistical and scientific evidence we know that the great majority of women can have spontaneous, complication-free deliveries. So why are there still so many interventions? Are we simply bullied because we're giving birth in the wrong surroundings? Are we brainwashed by outdated notions that it'll be too painful to bear and dangerous for the baby? Or has the medical system made us too comfortable, paranoid and reliant on aids? Probably all of these reasons, but the question we really need to ask ourselves is what effect this has on the future health and temperament of our children.

It's often been said that we're at a crucial point for humanity. How babies are born into this world may play a greater role than many people would like to believe. The primal period from gestation through birth and early infancy form the basis for our development, health and capacity to love. What can we do as mothers apart from being informed consumers? Is it enough to be more mindful about the choices we make? Maybe we need to start by demedicalizing our pregnancies and stop focusing on the potential problems. If birth is uninterrupted, babies are more likely to be born into a secure, loving environment. Once childbirth is understood in the spiritual context in which it actually belongs, we will have reached the next step in evolution and raised our awareness, and possibly the consciousness of the planet.

# CHAPTER 10

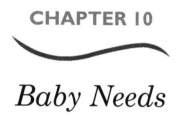

# *Baby Needs*

## THE BABYMOON

### *What to Do with a Baby?*

Once the excitement of birth has passed, it begins sinking in that you have an entirely new situation on your hands. A tiny, helpless bundle is reliant on you for absolutely *everything*, 24-uninterrupted-hours-of-the-day long. This can be overwhelming for even the most worldly-wise, efficient in every sense, done-it-all woman. Babies do not come complete with manuals, although you'll be surprised how suddenly everyone's a paediatrician, from your beloved mother-in-law to the mad granny down the road. Just as when you were pregnant, too much advice is confusing, and when you're feeling fragile it can make you feel downright inadequate. Let it drone right over that sleepy head of yours, because anything remotely useful will automatically be stored in your newly acquired mummy-hard drive. To avert ever so tiring arguments on basic life principles, just nod to everything suggested and let your common sense bin the spam.

It's not easy coping with know-it-alls, especially those from the outdated 'You'll spoil him, if you hold him' camp. To these heartless folk I just say, 'Let's continue this conversation once you've read some neuroscience.' Because when the door is firmly closed – keeping all the interferers out – the baby will be cared for perfectly well by the people who love it most in the world: mami and papi (those same people who will pay for any therapy costs should they really botch it up that badly).

In the first days and weeks you probably have lots of questions. There are countless sources for research, including your midwife (if you still trust her after the birth) and that thing called the internet – possibly the last place you have time to look right now. There are so many different theories, ideologies, fashions and approaches to baby-rearing, you're bound to get even more lost than you already feel. Eventually you'll find your own way and luckily you don't need a degree in child psychology to master the basics. Babies have very simple needs and these usually have to do with food and love.

## Smitten

Not all mothers bond with their babies straight away; so much depends on what kind of labour and birth you had and how soon you're able to recover. However, most mothers and fathers at some point in the first weeks fall in love big time with their new present. Getting besotted with your baby follows a simple law of nature that prevents us from eating our offspring, or at least remembering to take them home after a grocery shop. Compared to our mammal relatives, human babies are born the most helpless and dependent. Was this cunningly intended so that parents spend those first blurry weeks cradling and admiring their delicate progeny, feeling entirely responsible – and consequently loved up? If it's your first, you're highly susceptible to developing what

Mumsnet aptly calls 'Precious Firstborn Syndrome'. This involves displaying dubious behaviour such as spraying anyone who comes near your lambkin with industrial, hospital-grade disinfectant or rubbing baby shampoo directly into your own eyes to check if it stings.

Becoming a mum is the best thing in the world. The truth. Every day your heart fills up a little more with love. It's what's called unconditional love; a love so strong it will get you through them calling you nasty names, breaking your antique table, and teenage angst. Then, when they've eaten your food, spent all your money and left your house in a mess, they bugger off to live with a psycho. But you still love them because they're forever your little darling. That's just the dysfunctional way it is. It's not money that makes the world go round, it is parental love. Otherwise the planet would have been taken over by chipmunks long ago. All parents think their baby is the most special, beautiful (until you see photos later and realize you gave birth to Gollum) future candidate for the Nobel Peace Prize. And that's the way it should be.

## GROWING

It's remarkable just how fast babies grow; the first year sees huge leaps from a helpless little tiddly pooper who can't hold his own head up to a boisterous, curious pre-toddler determined to walk on two legs. Every baby is different, so no need to call the child psychologist if yours is lagging behind (or the talent scouts if she's in front). This part[1] is not to get you comparing – there will be plenty of competition from those trying to out-mum you wherever there's a swing or play mat. Anyway, it's hardly an entry ticket to Oxbridge if she can pincer-grip a penne at 3 months.

## *The First Month or So*

Depending on your baby's character and maturity at birth she will, over the course of the first weeks, start acknowledging the weird new world around her. She'll start recognizing sounds and turn her eyes in that direction – very exciting if this is mum or dad's voice; even more exciting when her neck muscles are strong enough for a slight turn of head to look over at you. Babies can also talk: they gurgle, coo, squeal and grunt with pleasure. Basic – and obviously baby-like – these sounds may be, but they are your offspring's first verbal communication attempts, so talk back. When she is able to fix your gaze, you will be able to communicate that way, too.

Over the course of a few weeks your baby will adjust her body clock and stay awake for longer periods of time – and thankfully asleep long enough for you to actually go to the loo. She's exploring the world, so stimulate her senses by singing to her, play chimes or dangle any object that makes a noise (yes, this is the stage where we can regress, too). She can't deliberately grab hold of anything yet, but her finger reflex means she'll grasp (so you can pretend she's holding things and take funny photos). Her other strong reflex is sucking, which those mothers who breastfeed will be feeling as well as seeing. At some point in this period all parents' most favourite thing can happen: your baby will smile, tentatively at first, maybe passing wind the second time, but eventually it will be at you. Bull's-eye, straight through the heart.

## *3 Months-ish*

Little bairn's character may start emerging more now as he becomes interested in what's one step beyond. He may be less grumpy and sleepy and keener to explore. Once your baby can hold his head steadily, he's mastered the important first milestone that leads to everything else like rolling, sitting, crawling and walking (hold on, not yet ...). This is a good time to regularly put him on his front, so he gains strength and can practise pushing up. You have to watch him carefully, though; gone are the days of putting him on a bed and expecting him to remain motionless. Many babies try out their first back-to-front roll the exact moment you decide to shampoo your hair. He will also start swiping at things (your nose, the rattle, his own fascinating foot) because he's gaining coordination and perspective of where he is and what's out there. Eagle-eyes is also starting to see better: he's no longer just tracking along edges, so you can introduce books with colourful pictures and start reading to him. Playing is becoming bags of fun so you can peek-a-boo, pat-a-cake and tickle-them-toes. Any of these games can result in parents' reward number two: the giggle. Your infant is the ultimate Zen master. This little enlightened guru fully understands what is actually real and 'The Power of Now' much better than any of us adults.

## Already Half a Year

Once her back muscles are strong enough and she has mastered balancing, little madam will be able to sit without support. This happens gradually as she figures out how to prop herself up with her arms in front of her, frog-like. She's likely to spend a lot of time enjoying her newly gained independence and upright perspective on the world. It also makes your daily life easier because you can forget the heavy baby paraphernalia and prop her up while you're trying on clothes in high-street shops (she may even give you advice). Most babies' two front upper teeth come through around 6 months, so expect a bit of soreness and even a raised temperature. It's the time when they have an urge to chew, putting everything into their mouths, preferably the dirty things. Remember she's building up her immune system, and a bit of muck is actually good for her. Cigarette butts are not so great, but for some reason babies always find them. Her hand control will have improved and she'll love grabbing things. She's also beginning to comprehend cause and effect hence her favourite game is dropping things and watching you pick them up. You can also have fun getting her to mimic sounds. She babbles away and might even sing along with you (like those people who pretend they know the words). She'll express attachment by holding out her arms for you to pick her up. She might even cry when you leave which is the beginning of separation anxiety. She's firmly understood that you are mum and can show that she really loves and needs you. Ah!

## Counting 9 Months

Adventurous babies will now try lunging forward and this leads to crawling on all fours. Once they can crawl on a flat surface, they look for the next challenge – crawling up stairs (crawling down, not so easy). However, some babies never crawl: some bottom shuffle, others tummy slither and some go straight to pulling up and walking. The main aim is being mobile. My parents say I tracked my intended path and then rolled myself from one corner of the room to another at high speed. Many babies will now also start pulling themselves up on anything that looks solid (but often isn't). They're strengthening their legs ahead of walking and will often cruise along holding onto furniture. Your copy-cat may also clap, wave or do the 'Red Indian' (wah-wah); these are great party tricks that guarantee entertainment for the visiting grandparents. Putting things into containers and unpacking are other favourite pastimes (fill treasure boxes in different places for the wee investigator) as well as opening and closing doors – miniatures and giant, real ones. He'll be able to inspect things with his pincer grasp; you'll be astounded how dexterous your little one has become when you find the contents of your jewellery box in the cat litter.

## *Happy Birthday*

Coming up to 1 year, many children will be able to walk holding onto your hands. Then when the courage, balance and strength are there, that milestone of a moment – your baby's first step – a joy-whooping, tear-jerking event for mum and dad. Hold off buying the mini Nikes, though; experts say going barefoot increases balance and coordination. You can get some soft cruisers for going outside if it's cold. Apart from mobile independence your child may now be able to drink from a sippy cup – by herself – and she's starting to express very clearly when she doesn't want something (not strapped into that pram again!). She'll defiantly assert herself and ignore you, not to incur your wrath, but simply because the world wants to be explored and the best way to do this is by touching and doing. As her higher cognitive abilities develop, she can reason and even make word-like sounds – 'mama' and 'dada' being the ultimate crowd-pleasers.

### YOUR BABY'S BRAIN

During the first 3 years, a baby's brain triples in weight and establishes billions of nerve connections. Babies have far more neural pathways than adults because they're constantly learning new things about their world. Adult neural pathways are like motorways compared to the thousands of interconnected lanes in babies' brains. Childhood is particularly long in humans, because you need that time to play and experiment and accumulate all the learning that makes you such an efficient grown-up. Babies' brains are very flexible – what neuroscientists call *plasticity* – in order to change and adapt to experiences. Key areas grow or shrink, depending on how they're used. The latest findings show that babies learn more, imagine more, care more and experience more than us *big oafs*. They're also much smarter than even we could have thought possible.[2]

## BONDING

### Home Alone

While some mothers find romance with their descendant through conversations in the womb, other women scrape through babyhood finding they can relate better once their child turns two (or nineteen and doing a physics degree). Affectionate feelings have a habit of increasing and growing with the baby, especially once you're less tired, out of the feeding-wiping poop loop and able to appreciate your child's emerging character. We have very high cultural expectations of motherhood, with lots of pressure in our nuclear family set-up to be the sole caretaker. So it's no wonder many women feel they're falling short. The immediate shock of switching from girl-about-town to being stuck home-alone with a needy, speechless dependant can be gigantic.

### Baby Boot Camp

Some women take to motherhood like ducks to sodden bread; some go with the flow not minding the chaos; some women panic that they're doing it all wrong. Like a good friend of mine who followed one of the bestselling 'routines' books (no names being mentioned) explained: 'I've turned to books all my life for information. I did 10 weeks of motherhood without guidance and was lost. I needed someone to spell it out to me. I just didn't have the confidence to trust my own instincts.' She did literally walk around with *the book* in her hands, as she got through the first months. My friend is on her second child now (at 41) and says she's done with 'the rules' because she's more chilled out. I'd say use whatever works for you and your baby. As long as there are parents with questions there will be books with answers.

## *Ways to Bond with Baby*

- Enjoy activities you can do together like *Baby and me yoga* or *Baby swimming*.
- Give your baby a massage – many local councils now offer free courses.
- Sing rhymes and silly songs with her.
- Kiss her nose, belly and feet – soon she'll kiss you back.
- Pull funny faces, tickle her and laugh with her.
- Look at picture books together.
- Do some exercises like leg-cycling, arm-waving and hold her upside-down (if she's a flexi-baby).
- Keep eye-contact as much as possible, especially when massaging or changing nappies.
- Splash around in the bath together.
- Put on your favourite music and dance with your baby in your arms or encourage her wiggle away to it.
- Let her lie, crawl or cruise around naked (preferably on a tiled floor or warm lawn if you're worried about 'spills').
- From about 6 months she'll love pans, pots, lids and other utensils – you can have a kitchen concert.
- She'll enjoy discovering things in boxes – put objects with different shapes, textures, colours and noises in a 'treasure chest' for her.
- Take her to a place with water: the river, lake or sea, and go on a boat.
- Hang out with some animals or go and see some she doesn't know yet, like park deer, farm animals and local elephants (you know, the ones who live at Number 19).

### WHY LOVE MATTERS

New understanding about how the brain works proves early experiences have a huge impact on future perceptions, choices and habits – they basically mould the brain. A baby is born needing social interaction and being able to recognize fear, anger and love in a facial expression or tone of voice. Latest research in neuroscience shows that the early relationship with caregivers affects future wellbeing.[3] Ample affection and interaction during the first years encourage good social skills. Scientists have also shown that feeling safe and cared-for leads to more neural connections in the brain and the later ability to deal with stress. Extreme cases, such as Romanian orphans left alone in their cots all day, had a 'virtual black hole where their orbito-frontal cortex should be';[4] meaning that their social skills were severely impaired.

## Positive Play

These findings have confirmed what attachment psychologists have been saying for decades. If a child sees relationships as a source of comfort and pleasure then this will help build his confidence and basic trust. Caregivers are encouraged to make a child feel worthy and secure, to listen to him, react to him, notice things, be responsive to his feelings, validate and take him seriously. This does not mean making him the centre of attention all the time. Childcare experts suggest letting him watch and join in with things you need to do. A child basically wants to learn from elders and have his discovery of the world supported. 'Finishing off' tasks for a child may be well-meaning and faster but it implies he can't do it. Too much negative reinforcement will make him grow up thinking that he's not good enough. Many child psychologists today suggest you turn negatives into positives. So, for example, you gently exchange the forbidden item for one that is allowed, or you firmly and confidently say, 'Let's do this instead,' or 'Look, Mummy's doing this' (kids love to copy). That way you can sneakily protect them from harm. Saying things like, 'Watch out, you'll fall' or 'Don't touch that you'll cut yourself,' creates negative expectations. The child will inevitably fulfil those expectations, based on his nature as a social being (and don't forget the Law of Attraction!). If you trust your child to follow his innate wisdom, he won't stumble over rocks. Have confidence in him; he's closer to instinct and less conditioned by fear than you are.

---

**NATIVE DISCIPLINE**

The Efe Pygmies of central Africa never tell their children how to behave, nor do they try to control them. The Belgian ethnologist Jean-Pierre Hallet, who lived with them for years, said he never saw a Pygmy adult hit or criticize a child. The children just copy what adults do and learn about danger without doing harm to themselves or their self-confidence. They learn by example and doing, rather than rewards and punishment.

---

## FEEDING

### Nursing Dilemmas

Breastfeeding is making a comeback in our culture after decades of being discouraged due to all sorts of screwed-up reasons and aggressive marketing campaigns by powdered milk corporations. Today nursing is still complex: on one hand it's encouraged by health authorities but at the same time women aren't assisted enough to persist with it. If every new mum is supposed to breastfeed (making all those who don't feel completely crap) then she needs to be supported from the very start; this includes:

•   Hospital and birthing centre staff respecting your wishes to breastfeed straight after birth and not taking the baby away at night to bottle-feed it.

- Breastfeeding professionals showing you how to do it in an understanding manner (remember, we're all hormonal after birth) and continuing to show you until you really get it – this can take weeks if you're having problems.
- Family members respecting your need for privacy ('Yes, Uncle John, those are my breasts').
- Society giving it the recognition it deserves (how about some comfy chairs in specially designated cordoned-off areas of public spaces? Or healthcare incentives such as 'massage vouchers' for each month you nurse?).

Many women these days don't or can't breastfeed properly because they're not supported by their environment, be it husbands, other mothers, where and how they gave birth, or jobs they have to do. Sometimes work gets in the way, making it a challenge to breastfeed exclusively for 6 months. Whatever you are able to do, it is so worth it.

## Liquid Gold

If you imagine the amount of milk a mother gives to her baby over the course of a few months and then think of that fluid in terms of energy, it's clear that breastfeeding is real work and a serious commitment. It takes up endless hours of your time while you're expected to fulfil your other responsibilities competently as well. It means you have to lay off the booze and bad habits without anyone patting you on the back. However, the sacrifice is peanuts compared to the rewards. No one can dispute the superior quality of breastmilk. It enhances the baby's immune system, protects against disease and reduces the risk of allergies. Exclusive breastfeeding reduces infant mortality caused by common illnesses such as diarrhoea or pneumonia, and encourages a speedy recovery. Long-term studies showed breastfed children grew into taller, more intelligent, healthier adults with fewer weight issues and lower risk of heart disease, asthma, allergies and diabetes.

Apart from the huge health benefits, you're giving your child a fundamental feeling of security; setting him up for life and promoting his sensory and cognitive development. Breastmilk is also free, easy to digest, convenient, portable, comes out at the perfect temperature and doesn't involve faffing around sterilizing bottles or mixing formula powder. Another pleasant side effect is that it doesn't make your baby's poo stink like formula milk does. Nursing has been proven to help you recover better after birth, protect you against breast cancer, ovarian cancer, heart disease, diabetes and stroke (if you persist with it long enough). And, mostly importantly, it's the easiest, fastest and most long-lasting way to bond with your baby.

The first few days after your baby is born your breasts are not producing milk but *colostrum*. Colostrum is a brilliant stroke of Mother Nature because it tastes similar to amniotic fluid. The thick, sticky elixir contains millions of immune-active cells that can neutralize the most dangerous microbes and infections. This is vitally important because inside the womb there wasn't a single germ. Colostrum forms the basis for healthy intestinal flora and contains enormous amounts of fatty acids – the key components for brain development.

At around day four your milk will come in, so this is when the feeding party should start if you want to avoid painful, engorged breasts. Hopefully you'll have an ecstatic baby who greedily drinks until she's drunk, stoned and delirious. Apart from the antibodies mentioned above, breastmilk has all the vital nutrients in the right quantities. As the baby grows, your milk miraculously changes according to her nutritional and calorific needs. Feel-good endorphins and love hormones are passed through the milk to the child, something that formula milk can never emulate.

## SOME MILKY FACTS

The World Health Organization and UNICEF both suggest mothers should breastfeed their infants exclusively for 6 months (no additional food, drink or water). Thereafter, breastmilk provides half the necessary nutrients from 6 months to 1 year of age, and infants should receive complementary foods with continued breastfeeding up to 2 years and beyond.

Sweden has a 98 per cent rate of exclusive breastfeeding for the first 4 months – the highest level in the world (*quelle surprise*, the country with long periods of maternity *and* paternity leave). Some 53 per cent of women continue breastfeeding for 6 months or longer. Norway comes in a close second (also a country with good maternity/paternity packages).

A study in the US focusing on women who breastfed over 12 months found that greater age, education and exclusive breastfeeding led to a longer duration of nursing.[5]

A US cost analysis study estimates that nearly 900 babies could be saved each year, along with billions of dollars, if 90 per cent of women breastfed their babies exclusively for the first 6 months, preventing hundreds of deaths and childhood illnesses.[6]

Scientific analysis of human fossils over a million years old found in Atapuerca, Spain showed that breastmilk was the principal form of food for the first 3 to 4 years of age. Scientists concluded this led to good health for the rest of their lives.[7]

## Getting the Knack

In terms of starting out, the most important thing you need to know is: feed the baby as much as you can (think farm animal!) for the first weeks. Basically the more you feed, the more milk you make. There will be days of feeding frenzy and days when your baby is sleepy. Don't worry too much about routines; they will come automatically later once your milk supply is established.

'What do they say? Twenty minutes each side every 4 hours?
Bollocks! More like 8–18 times a day for the first 5 to 6 weeks,
and that 24/7.'
**ENTRY IN MY DIARY, AUGUST 2008**

Try not to miss any feeds, because replacing with formula or 'topping up' with bottles is the fastest way to diminish your own supply. Your breasts won't be getting the right messages to produce more milk. It's really not worth obsessing about feeding duration, ounces of weight gain or the whole foremilk/hindmilk debate. It varies from woman to woman, but generally milk starts off thin to quench the baby's thirst and then, as the flow slows down, it turns into the high-calorie thick stuff. Genius! Your baby may empty one breast and then fall asleep halfway through the second (which is why it's a good idea to burp him every so often). You can more or less alternate which breast you start him on, so that both sides are equally stimulated. But as long as your baby has wet nappies, is nursing regularly and growing, there's no need to change anything, time your feeds or introduce any formula.

If you're finding it difficult to breastfeed because you have sore or cracked nipples, it could be because the baby isn't latching on properly. Make sure your baby fills his mouth with the areas around your nipple, not just the nipple itself (dummies teach babies poor latches, so avoid one if you can). You also need to hold him close to your breast, at the right angle. Look at diagrams and photos to get some ideas. You can rub your own milk on sore breasts after feeds to heal them (before you have to revert to sticking cabbage leaves in your bra). Don't give up trying; most problems can be resolved. An independent midwife or kind breastfeeding advisor may be able to help you.

## CAN'T DO

My gynaecologist says there's no such thing as a woman who *can't* breastfeed. Forty years of data from The Farm Midwifery Center proves that 99 per cent of mothers were able to breastfeed. Nursing is actually something older mothers do more easily, due to being well informed and having the time and determination.

## *Easy Peasy*

After a while on the game – and you've got through a fair share of breast pads/bed sheets/t-shirts with those lactic eruptions – you may want to try expressing. It's no picnic getting to grips with the wacky let-down reflex, but mama's-homebrew-in-a-bottle will give you a couple of hours off to catch up with girlfriends/ the latest film/a few hours' kip while doting daddy – or lovely babysitter – do the bonding.

Most experts advise against using a bottle too soon or frequently because it can make the baby a bit lazy at the breast.

If and when you have to leave your baby for longer periods due to that other duty outside of the home they also call 'work', then expressing can be a way to prolong breastfeeding. Many working mothers find nursing to be very flexible, feeding – and reconnecting with their child – when they get home in the evening, first thing in the morning and fully breastfeeding at the weekend or days off. The US study I mentioned earlier showed that 68 per cent of those who breastfed longer than a year returned to work before their infant was a year old.

## *Mobile Feeding*

I found nursing the most relaxing (and least distracting for a naturally curious baby) in a comfortable, private place. It's a good idea to prepare a corner of your home with cushions, books, magazines and a big jug of water or herbal tea (now that you fully comprehend the concept *dying of thirst*). The midwives where I gave birth told me to copy how tribal South American and African women lactate, on the go. As soon as I got the hang of breastfeeding lying down and sitting, I started walking and found this to be very practical. It means you can get on with what want to do while your infant simultaneously fulfils his needs. It may sound a bit too 'earth mother' for your liking but believe me this is the best way for a busy, modern woman to manage her duties.

A front-carrier or hammock sling is perfect for breastfeeding: your hands are free, you can nurse without anyone noticing and your baby can feed and sleep as he wishes. This is what I call *being in the flow* with your child and your life.

## *Breast-fixated*

In our neck of the woods there are some repressed, warped beliefs on full-term breastfeeding (often wrongly labelled 'extended breastfeeding'). In many Asian countries infants are nursed until they're ready to wean themselves, and they certainly aren't 'too attached' to their mums, nor do the mothers' breasts 'droop'. I was horrified to read some ridiculous advice in a popular baby-care book which said that if a woman is concerned about her body image it's best for her *not* to breastfeed!! So, just to make this clear: your breasts DON'T sag if you breastfeed, nor does longer breastfeeding wear them down. Big fluctuations in weight and ill-supporting bras during pregnancy are to blame for loss of elasticity, if anything. Neither I, nor any of my friends who breastfed, noticed much of a change; your breasts just return to their pre-pregnancy size and shape when you're done. Since the dawn of time breasts were designed for feeding babies; then someone along the line bagged them for selling stuff because good profit could be made.

The allure of bosoms is that they fulfil dual purposes. They are both nurturing and erotic; they produce life-fluid and pleasure, comfort and excitement. So use them!

## *Your Food to Feed*

If you're breastfeeding exclusively, you don't need to worry that your baby's getting enough or good enough milk from you. Breastmilk always has the perfect composition to fulfil your infant's needs, and do this consistently. Studies show that the balance of nutrients does not change dramatically if your diet is lacking. However, you do need to watch vitamins A, $B_6$ and calcium as there is an increased need for these. You might become weaker and more tired if you're not eating properly. You should also remember that toxins do go straight to the milk so eating an organic, whole-food diet is still recommended.

## *Needed Extras*

- Drink lots of water (add a pinch of Himalayan or unprocessed sea salt once a day) and herbal teas; make your own green power juice (with, for example, spinach or broccoli with apple) and fruit smoothies. Producing milk will dehydrate you, so aim to drink at least 3 litres between meals.
- Get extra protein from sprouts such as lentils, chick peas, mung beans.
- You need 550 mg more calcium daily. Find it in green vegetables like broccoli, seaweeds and the superfood, maca.
- Include oils such as cold-pressed olive and flaxseed oil, and don't forget your omega 3, whether you supplement or eat oily fish.
- Eat broccoli, spinach and carrots for vitamin A, bananas for $B_6$, yeast flakes for B vitamins (the whole world is B-deficient right now), molasses for iron and calcium.

- Bee pollen has all the body's essential vitamins and minerals.
- Snack on sesame, pumpkin and sunflower seeds (soaked for about an hour in water for easier digestion) for zinc and calcium. Spread tahini on toast or veg.

---

**FOOD FOR THOUGHT**

After 7 years of living off light or pranic energy, a Brazilian woman gave birth to her naturally conceived seventh child at age 51. She has successfully breastfed her healthy daughter for 15 months,[8] despite not eating since 2001. Doreen Virtue, a clairvoyant metaphysician and author who gives angel readings, says: 'Humans are evolving to become less dependent on eating for energy and nourishment. First we'll become vegetarians, then raw foodists and drink only juice until we finally become "breatharians", receiving our nutrition from the prana life-force in the air. All this will help us adapt to Earth's changing food supplies as we get away from processed foods and move toward harvesting fresh produce.'[9]

---

## *Lotta Bottle*

If you're not breastfeeding or you start introducing formula milk before 6 months, you'll need to choose a suitable variety. Of course you know me by now – I'd go for the least mass-produced, most organic version (in a benzyl-free or glass bottle). Formulas all have to conform to Government standards and some will include pro-biotics or essential fatty acids. Cow's milk consumption in infants is linked to diabetes and other health issues, apart from it containing hormones that could be problematic. Goat's-milk formula is closer to breastmilk and better tolerated by those who are susceptible to allergies or congestion. Avoid soy-based formulas because soya can draw calcium from the bones, and contains hormones that seem unsuitable for male children especially. A recent analysis showed the most popular brands of infant formula to contain very high traces of aluminium contamination, particularly products containing soya or designed for babies who are lactose intolerant.[10]

## *Weaning*

If you listened to others (granddad, for example) you would give your baby a sausage and a beer at 4 months, but the general consensus is that solids shouldn't be introduced before 6 months. Why? Lots of reasons: the digestive tract isn't closed yet, the pancreas isn't ready, the kidneys are immature, the digestive enzymes aren't developed, there's a risk of obesity and allergies ... anyway why would you be bothered with the added hassle? If your baby is happy with milk alone, there's no need to hurry.

There are two main schools of thought when it comes to weaning: spoon-feeding purees and mash or baby-led weaning which involves your kid munching – or gumming – his way through finger foods. Think more along the lines of cucumber sticks than the canapés you soak up with wine at parties.

You can prepare some scrumptious healthy snacks for babies with a bit of inspiration and nutritional know-how. The best time to introduce solid foods is just before breast- or bottle-feeding. Build up gradually, introducing one new food at a time to see how well your baby tolerates it.

Another general guideline is no gluten, eggs, meat, fish, peanuts, honey or cow's milk for the first year. After 6 months you can introduce raw, organic goat's milk or yoghurt. Pure coconut milk is a great alternative – this is the closest thing in nature to breastmilk because it's the only other food that contains lauric acid. Remember, babies still need at least 600 ml of milk daily up to 9 months, and 400 ml thereafter until they are a year old. I was also a little fundamentalist about banning salt and sugar; babies' tiny livers can't cope with salt, and sugar, well, it's simply to avoid the hyperactive tantrums and rotten teeth. And here's another warning: research conducted at Cardiff University found that children who eat sweets daily are more likely to be violent as adults.[11]

Please note that this is a chapter in your life where all designer clothes and other items you're particularly fond of should be kept at the very back of your wardrobe and under no circumstances worn around your baby. You'll have goo dribbled over your leg, porridge smeared on your front and remainders of root vegetables permanently stuck to your right shoulder (or the shoulder where you most hold your child).

## GETTING AROUND

### Baby Outings

It's really good for your baby to get out of the house for some oxygen and vitamin D; it's vital for mum's sanity to change scenery and maybe talk to another adult. Everything is stimulating to a new baby, so you needn't do anything baby-specific. Enjoy this time to do what YOU want, be it meeting a friend, taking a walk or getting a spray-tan (well, maybe not quite). There'll be plenty of years when you're stuck with 'soft play centres' and child-friendly/ adult-heinous activities. Until your baby can crawl or cruise it'll be peasy, so make the most of these low-maintenance months.

However, you do need to be well prepared. It's not like those pre-mum days when you popped out freshly showered with a carefully made-up face, well-put-together outfit, your wallet in hand and keys in pocket. No, this is far more complicated. You have another little person who does uncontrollable things like poo and dribble and vomit at the most inappropriate moments. Your bag (be it the latest nappy-changing satchel, a stylish Cath Kidston hold-all or a Lake District-worthy rucksack) needs to be pre-packed; the easiest way is to *keep* it packed and then stock up what's missing.

Once you have all the nappies, wipes, muslins, bibs, toys, bottles, baby snacks and changes of clothing, you need to dress pint-size for going outside. And she's very likely to choose this opportunity to soil her nappy, which means you have to start the dressing procedure all over again. Then you need to find your phone, which you left in the kitchen, or was it the toilet? Having grabbed yourself any old coat and put on last season's shoes, your poor child is overheated but luckily she can't punch you yet, so off you go. Finally out of the door you realize your keys are in another jacket and your wallet somehow doesn't seem to be in your bag either. You also haven't had time to put any mascara on. But you fully comprehend why they say mothering's selfless.

## Picking that Pram

At some point you'll probably want to invest in a pram – this is a useful item for putting your shopping in while you focus on calming a fussy baby (someone should tell supermarkets to dim those lights). When choosing your model it's a good idea to take your child for a test drive, inside the shop, because she will, after all, be the vehicle's main passenger. You'll want to check out suspension, wheels (are they robust, can they swivel?), handle height, space for essential day-luggage and, most importantly, ease of folding. There's nothing more manic that getting on a moving bus with a pram that won't collapse and a wriggling infant. Ideally you should be able to fold it up one-handed – so you have the other free to stop wild one from running under the bus. Another very important – often overlooked – point is whether it fits into the boot of your car and is it light enough to carry? I personally think it's vital for the pram or buggy to have the fully reclined option so baby can doze while you chat away in coffee shops. Also remember, newborns can't sit up yet.

Cunning shop assistants may try to coax you into buying the bank-breaking *travel system*. I find these a complete waste of money, plastic and space because you can only use the *car seat* and *cot* sections for the first months (when it's nicer to carry babies anyway). After that they want to sit up, so you really just need a lightweight, foldable, practical stroller. However, some mothers swear by the ergonomically designed, lie-down pushchairs and have the budget to get these short-life Ferraris. One last word of warning; do beware of the stroller wars in your local park – they can get ugly.

## Travelling Far with Baby

This can be as easy or hard as you make it. A lot depends on how adventurous your travels were before munchkin came along, but generally wherever you go, a baby can follow, especially a non-wriggling infant under a year old. Toddlers will want to run around on planes and talk to everyone on the bus/train/hovercraft, so travelling with a baby really is a piece of cake by comparison (or maybe just training for what comes later). The first rule is: arrive early, because things always take longer with a baby. Make sure your child stays well hydrated (milk or water) and that you have an extra blanket. Bring some toys and books for entertainment and enough nappies, wipes, snacks and changes of clothing for the trip. If you're going somewhere remote you may want to pack extra nappies and baby food in your suitcase. Don't pack too many baby clothes because you can always find a place to rinse them. It won't be the kind of *holiday* you might be used to, but *being elsewhere* with an infant can be lots of fun.

## Baby Wearing

Out of all the baby accessories I have, nothing has been more practical or frequently used than my baby sling/carrier (all three of them). A good substitute for tired arms, the bouncy seat, playpen, cot and pram, you can walk, sit and feed your baby in it. You can cook while your baby sleeps in it (on your back, preferably), hoover and clean, fold the laundry, run errands, jump on and off buses, walk ALL those stairs in Tube corridors and soothe a fussing baby. A baby sometimes cries when it's over-stimulated, so you can use a sling to protect it from the outside world or just rock it gently to sleep; the rhythm of walking and hearing mum's heartbeat is very 'womb-like'. If you prefer using the pram, it's still a good idea to take a sling with you for moments when the baby can't be soothed (and you don't have time to sit down and do it). Even for toddlers a good sturdy baby carrier – where your child sits on your back – is ideal to whip out when they get too tired to walk. There are some you fasten around the waist to take the weight off your shoulders (and they don't look remotely *hippy*). Carrying a heavy child – if you do it correctly – is actually good for strengthening your bones and preventing osteoporosis. For part of the year we run a beach yoga resort in Goa, so carrying my son in a sling is the only way to move around. No pram – no matter how much of a Hummer-tank replica – could four-wheel drive across those mounds of sand.

## The Continuum Concept

This idea, based on evolutionary human development, says that to become happy adults, babies require the kind of nurturing as practised by our ancient relatives. After spending years in the South American jungle among native peoples, the author and psychotherapist Jean Liedloff wrote a book to share her observations. The Yequana tribe carry their babies in slings as they go about their daily business, be it walking, running or canoeing. Babies are stimulated to experience and learn about the world from the safety of being *in arms*. Liedloff noticed that babies never cried, slept when they were tired and had no tension in their bodies like many Western infants. Their bodies were supple and relaxed, and they were able to discharge excess energy via a dynamic, moving caregiver. When they started crawling and walking babies were trusted to explore by their parents and they would come back for reassurance if needed. The Yequanas believe that human nature is good and so only expect good things from their children. Liedloff concluded that the way we often treat babies in Western society is not appropriate for our species and is the cause of widespread alienation, neurosis and unhappiness.

## SLEEPING

### Newborn Slumber

I know you're likely to be tired, but this section is about your baby (your qualms will be dealt with in the next chapter). There are many sons of man (and daughters of woman), so if you have a baby who sleeps through the night at 6 weeks, then that is wonderful – just don't shout about it, you might get struck by a deranged, sleep-deprived mother falling out of a tree (well, stranger things have happened). Fact is, most babies don't – and won't – sleep through the night for a good few months. I never said motherhood was for wimps, so don't start packing your bags now.

At first babies know no difference between day and night. Then, hopefully soon – thanks to your gentle guidance, good example and feeding cues – they adapt by waking and eating more during daylight hours, giving everyone in the house a few hours' rest. A good rule of thumb:

- Day = noise, light, stimulating activities
- Night = quiet, dark, boring.

Newborns will nap pretty much anywhere, so you can go about your business – but remember they will sleep longer and better on a flat surface than in a car seat or baby bouncer.

There are basically three options for nights:

1. Sharing your bed – our cousins across the Atlantic have dubbed this 'co-sleeping'
2. Putting your baby down in a cot/crib/moses basket
3. Mix and match.

Many parents in the UK today have the cot by their bed in the first months and end up co-sleeping for part of the night due to exhaustion and simply because it is most convenient for breastfeeding (and better for the milk supply because the hormone prolactin is produced at night). It also means you have 24-hour surveillance and access to that little breathing nose when you wake up in a hot *is-she-still-alive?* sweat. Lying next to a caregiver has a calming effect: babies' heart rates have been found to synchronize with that of their mother, muscular activity is relaxed and breathing deepens. You won't, by the way, crush your baby (unless you're a drunk or druggie) because your sleeping body is attuned to your baby's whereabouts. Studies that monitored sleeping mother–infant pairs found them to be highly responsive to each other's movement; babies would breastfeed more but rarely cry.[12] It was concluded that mothers got at least as much, if not more sleep than those who slept without their babies.

A baby who wakes up hungry in (or near) the mother's bed will generally grunt, root around for the breast, suckle and then doze off back to the land of zzz; so will mum (even if she's bottle-feeding, hopefully). What's more comforting and likely to induce sleep than being close to your source of food and protection, and knowing it will be there when you wake up? Most of the citizens of planet Earth co-sleep in their little family cocoons; it is basically our modern, Western culture that has the money and space to give each member a separate cubicle. You can also try bringing the baby into bed to feed and then putting her back in her cot when she's sleeping – just make sure you change any dirty nappies beforehand, so as not to disrupt her.

This co-sleeping/sleeping nearby arrangement doesn't suit everyone; you might need your water-bed to yourself, your husband may get jealous, the cat usually sleeps with you and snores too loudly – whatever your set-up, I'd say traipsing all the way to the west wing to find a distraught, crying child and sitting up for hours to feed in a cold room while deliriously watching some garbage on cable TV is what leads to serious sleep deprivation. Mainstream childcare advice is to sleep with the baby in the same room or within earshot in the first months. Newborns have no concept of time or space or that they are no longer attached to you. So even if you were there just 2 minutes ago stroking his forehead, once you're gone, in the baby's mind you don't exist and he's alone to fend for himself. It's stressful for a helpless baby to be separated from the person who's supposed to keep him alive.

## Gentle 'Sleep Associations'

At some point parents start introducing what are commonly known as 'bedtime rituals'. These usually involve a bit of down-time or quiet playing time with dimmed lights to get the infant settled, a round of story-time (a book or five), cuddling and maybe a lullaby. For this you can whip out mothering tool number one – play those songs or sing those mantras you did during pregnancy; your baby will recognize them. The idea is that repetition and sleep associations will (eventually) cue your baby to know it is sleep time, and to look at bedtime as a lovely, safe place to be.

It's sensible to let someone else share the honour of bedtime rituals. You wouldn't want to deprive daddy of that, would you?

(Or deprive yourself of the start of every single programme on TV worth watching – and there aren't many.) Fathers may have a different way of doing things – he probably won't want to sing those mantras, for a start (well, who'd honestly want to listen?). Let your partner use his own technique, it will build up his fathering confidence, cement the bond with his child and give you more time off. If he refuses to help, you have my permission to fire him.

## Bad Habits Bollocks

I'd like to spend a moment addressing concerns about babies acquiring bad habits. First of all, you can't *spoil* a baby in the first year or two because she has no ego and simply isn't manipulative (except maybe Damian from *The Omen*). This notion that a baby – the purest version of human nature that exists – is expected to be *bad* is exactly where we've lost the plot (and some of those child-rearing 'experts' misled generations). All the 'don't go to her when she cries/succumb to her whims/give in to her/pander to her' doctrines have finally been proved wrong by neuroscientists and psychologists.

Interestingly enough the latest research confirms what our more primitive ancestors instinctively knew. Newborns are innately sociable, eager to adapt and reliant on responsive caregivers to meet their needs for immediate survival.

Babies are babies for such a short time and then they grow out of 'baby-ish' behaviour. So for those who say 'He'll get used to you holding him and then you'll never be able to put him down,' yeah, right! Try holding a wriggling, fidgeting toddler on your lap for more than 2 minutes – 'Oh, he just didn't grow out of being held,' 'I held him too much as a baby and now he doesn't want to run and play.' Or what about the common warning: 'If you let her sleep in your bed, she'll pick up bad habits'? All babies, at some point, realize that they're no longer part of your body and that you won't disappear overnight. They also grow out of sleeping in a cramped bed and want their own space (they start kicking you, lying crosswise and hogging the best part of the mattress – clearly demonstrating 'I need my own space' behaviour). By sleeping in your bed a baby is actually picking up *good* sleeping habits (night-time = quiet + everybody sleeping). The kids I know who are in their parents' bed age seven are the ones who never did it when they were babies.

A child basically has different needs which change as she grows. Mainstream psychology believes that if a need isn't satisfied in the relevant phase, it will crop up later in life as unfulfilled and the child will aim to recoup what she didn't have. So, basically: fulfil needs at the relevant time and you won't have a problem. In the natural scheme of life we start off as highly dependent and clingy and go through a process of learning and detaching, until we're fully independent. Why are parents so obsessed with hurrying up this process, or controlling how it unfolds? Another fact: we're the only animals on the planet who are systematically cruel to their newborn – separating infants from mothers at birth, leaving babies to cry, kicking them out of the warm family nest. And then we wonder why modern society is so dysfunctional and violent.

## CRYING

From now – until eternity probably – you'll react to a baby crying. Even if it's in the next carriage on the Northern Line (and your child is actually already going to college) you will, in that first heart-wrenching fraction of a second, think it's your baby. And that it is your responsibility to soothe those tears. This is the way motherhood rewires us.

The big disadvantage with being born unable to articulate clearly is the limitation in communicating needs; this is why babies cry. Once she's a bit older she'll find other ways to tell you what's up, be it pulling faces or pointing and babbling – a similar guessing game with a new set of rules.

## Why Baby Might Be Crying

*Hungry:* This is the most common reason a baby will cry. It's very clever, because crying will trigger your milk supply. Other signs of being hungry are if she sucks her fingers, makes sucking movements with her mouth, roots for the breast or wriggles her arms and legs. These cries are usually short and rhythmic.

*Tired:* A newborn is likely to receive lots of attention, which can be too much stimulation. Sometimes crying is simply her saying she's had enough and wants to rest. Take her to a quiet, dark place and try to settle her. Cries can be consistent and piercing. A lull in activity, losing interest, fussing, rubbing eyes, looking glazed and yawning can all be signs of tiredness in a slightly older baby.

*Uncomfortable:* She may be too hot or too cold. You can check by feeling her tummy or neck (hands and feet are usually cold anyway). She needs one more layer than you and no hat indoors. You can also check whether her clothes are too tight or itchy. She may have a dirty nappy.

*Gassy:* After all that milk she's glugged, your baby needs winding. Spend at least 5 minutes with her upright, patting her back. Trapped wind can be very painful and the huge burp that comes out will be a relief to both of you.

*Sick:* If the crying – which may be high-pitched and urgent – is accompanied by diarrhoea, vomiting or dry nappies, your baby might be ill. Being unusually quiet with these symptoms could also be a sign. If you think it's serious, give your doctor a call.

*Lonely:* Some babies need constant physical contact for comfort. He was inside your womb for 9 months, after all, where his needs were constantly met. Get a sling and carry him while you do other things.

*Teething:* This can start at around 3 months; signs are crying, gnawing, dribbling, red cheeks, mild fever (which can shoot up sporadically), smelly poo, nappy rash and diarrhoea. Give your baby something cold to chew on, try homeopathic Chamomilla; some mothers swear by amber necklaces.

*Colic:* Although it's not clear what causes it, inconsolable crying for at least 3 hours a day (usually in the evening) at least 3 days a week is often put down to colic. Signs may be your baby pulling up his legs in agony or passing lots of wind. There's no miracle cure – over-the-counter medicines aren't known to help – but it generally goes away at 3 months. Some experts say you should avoid cow's milk and citrus fruit if you're breastfeeding and drink camomile or aniseed tea. Cranial therapy can really help. You can also try walking around with your baby face-down along your forearm (tiger-in-the-tree hold) massaging him, or carrying him upright in a sling. The digestive system of a newborn is still being formed, so dealing with milk can be extremely painful. One school of thought says colic is just the baby telling us about his birth. Another says that colic comes from excessive tension in a baby who needs to be touched more.

## Other Things to Try

- Put on some calming music.
- Start the washing machine, hairdryer or hoover (I'm not joking, think womb: white noise and steady rhythm).
- Swaddle your baby in a soft blanket.
- Walk around with him in a sling, patting his bottom.

- Run, skip and jump around with him (this according to 'continuum concept' ideas).
- Rock him and yourself in a rocking chair.
- Massage his tummy.
- Let him suck on something.
- Sing your pregnancy mantras.
- Let someone else try to soothe him.
- Take deep breaths.
- Have a glass of wine (a small one if you're breastfeeding).

## CRANIAL OSTEOPATHY AND CRANIO-SACRAL THERAPY

Babies who cry a lot, babies with colic, babies who aren't feeding or sleeping properly, babies who have suffered complicated births and caesarean babies can all benefit from cranial therapy. This is very gentle application of pressure to the baby's head, neck, spine, pelvis and body to release tension and rebalance the flow of cranio-sacral fluid. Therapists are highly trained, but look for one who specializes in babies and children. Some experts believe *all* babies should see an osteopath to adjust any minor misalignments as early as possible.

## Crying It Out

Modern science may have found an answer to the endless debate between childcare experts on whether 'sleep training' is harmful: there is a measurable increase in the levels of stress hormones, pain-like sensations and disruption of temperature in a baby who's left to cry. According to psychotherapist Sue Gerhardt: 'Stress in infancy – such as consistently being ignored when you cry – is particularly hazardous because high levels of cortisol in the early months of life can also affect the development of other neurotransmitter systems whose pathways are still being established.'[13] Because a baby is born without the capacity to regulate himself or manage stress, he is dependent on an adult to maintain his cortisol levels. There is very little he can do but cry louder until he becomes so exhausted that he gives up and withdraws mentally. Numerous studies and cases have shown that babies who suffer extreme or repeated stress have either lower or higher than normal cortisol levels later in life. They also display a pattern of neural pathways and sensitivity of body cells that makes them react more strongly to difficulties. This puts them at a disadvantage when it comes to dealing with and recovering from stress. Consequences included reaching higher states of anxiety more quickly, depression or violent behaviour.

## HEALTH

A sick baby can turn the most composed parent into a headcase. It's obvious why: the possibility that a raised temperature indicates an incurable disease unknown to modern medicine crosses every parent's anxious mind. Plus you would easily rather be pinned down and have your eyelashes extracted with pliers than see your child suffer. However, babies do get ill; they also fall, bang their heads and sometimes they get fevers that bring on terrifying convulsions. The hard job for you is distinguishing between 'a bit unwell' and a genuine emergency. To prevent showing up at A&E for a blister (and them calling you needlessly hysterical), try consulting the numerous health encyclopaedias piled up on your bedside table and the internet first. Parents become very good at diagnosing problems because they know their babies better than anyone else. Saying that, I hope you have a wonderful GP with a wealth of practical knowledge who answers your calls with patient, sound advice even outside office hours.

The following are some easy cures. For the more serious stuff you're going to have to turn elsewhere.

## Home Remedies

*Bruises and bangs:* Arnica cream, oil or globules. However, any severe knocks to the head should be carefully observed, especially if your child vomits or his pupils change. In this case don't let him nap until you've seen a doctor.

*Bunged-up nose:* Use a snot extractor (oh the fun you'll have!). If it's dried-up snot you can put some breastmilk in a dropper, trickle some into each nostril to moisten the membranes and wash out the mucus.

*Conjunctivitis:* This eye infection is very common in newborns. Clean with distilled water and cotton wool, then, if you are able, put some breastmilk in each eye, as it contains the best antibodies you can find. If you're not breastfeeding use a few drops of colloidal silver.

*Common cold:* Give lots of fluids and use a humidifier or steam bath to ease breathing.

*Cough:* Put some raw onion slices on a plate near her bed to help break up thick, congested coughs. For a watery, tickly cough, put some lemon slices near a radiator or make a throat wrap. You can also add eucalyptus or pine oil to a bowl of water and, if she's over 6 months, add 2 drops of each to some vegetable oil and massage her chest.

*Cuts and grazes:* You can disinfect with tea tree oil or colloidal silver and then use a calendula-based cream for healing.

*Diarrhoea:* If you're breastfeeding, make sure your baby drinks even more. If she's eating solids, give her some rice goo or sticky rice and plenty of fluids.

*Fever:* Cool your baby down by removing clothes, give him a tepid bath and lots of liquids. You can try putting him in socks soaked in vinegar (yep!). Temperature is the body's way of fighting infection (bugs can't survive a raised temperature). However if it doesn't go down or is unreasonably high, give him baby paracetamol or baby ibuprofen – you can alternate. These will upset your baby's stomach so don't be surprised when he has diarrhoea. If your baby is under 3 months seek medical advice. If the fever persists or is very raised, seek medical advice.

*Head lice:* Put about 5 or 6 drops of tea tree oil in your usual baby shampoo and use a good lice comb. You can also try 'suffocating' the lice with olive oil.

*Mild burn:* Keep the affected area in a bowl of cool water (not cold or iced) for at least 10–20 minutes. Then you can apply aloe vera or lavender oil.

*Nappy rash:* Change wet nappies regularly, let his bottom air so that he's naked as often as possible; try calendula cream or a zinc oxide barrier cream.

*Vomiting:* Offer liquids and crackers if he's on solids, *Nux vom* homeopathic pills can help; breastfeed or offer liquids as much as possible. NB: If your child is refusing to eat for long, is lethargic or has dry nappies, you should get him checked for dehydration.

### HEALING ELIXIR

A huge number of diseases can be cured by simply sipping water containing suspended particles of silver.[14] Trials found that colloidal silver killed 650 harmful parasites and bacteria within 6 minutes. Unlike regular antibiotics, colloidal silver has no bad side effects and is completely non-toxic, which makes it safe for pregnant women and babies to use. Colloidal silver can also be used to overcome infections and repair a weakened immune system. It's cheap and easy to make this kind of water yourself by electrically charging colloids of pure silver in water. A wide variety of kits is available on the internet. The sale of colloidal silver water has now been banned in the EU, simply because silver has been patented after companies discovered what an amazing healer it is.

## *Just a Little Prick*

Vaccination is a rather contentious subject and another of the very difficult choices you have to make as a parent. When you were young you probably had about 10 injections. Most children today receive around 36 different routine injections before the age of 6, and if you count the individual vaccines it's about 50. Many experts – even those who believe in vaccinations – are against this blanket approach and question the safety of the complex vaccine schedules, in particular the combined or multiple injections, such as MMR (measles/mumps/Rubella).

Small babies' brains and nervous-system tissues are going through a period of rapid growth and development; this means they are particularly vulnerable to cellular and inflammatory damage. It is a universally recognized principle of toxicology that combinations of toxins increase the toxicity exponentially. Mercury has been getting the most attention because it's known to disturb the central nervous system and cause brain or neuro-degeneration. But aluminium – and other substances – added to most vaccines to boost immunity also increase toxicity and can accumulate in the brain. Then there is the issue of vaccine contamination through impurities, bacterial and viral fragments, and the impossibility of adequately controlling the manufacture of vaccines.

Another complex subject we are learning more about daily is immunology. It takes about 3 years for babies to develop their immune systems; a multiple viral jab can have an immuno-suppressive effect: so-called immune paralysis.

If you want to talk about evidence-based facts, there are no long-term, controlled randomized studies showing the safety or non-specific effects of today's combination of vaccines. But there is plenty of clinical and scientific data proving the risks. There is an undoubted link between the introduction of the current vaccine programme (36 jabs which start at a very young age) and the abrupt rise in autism, as well as ADD (attention deficit disorder) and other neurological and cognitive disorders. There are also too many accounts (and lawsuits) from parents who had a changed child after vaccination – be it an autoimmune disease or the triggering of autism after an MMR jab.

Read up on all the research before you decide. Think about each vaccine individually; which one is effective, what do we know about potential side effects, is the disease life-threatening or relevant to where you live? Don't forget that vaccines copy infections in order to create antibodies but they cannot create life-long immunity. If you're breastfeeding you can postpone vaccinating – until you've trawled through the volumes of information – because your baby will get her immunity through you. Many pro-vaccine experts even recommend waiting until the baby has passed the key phase for brain development. You really shouldn't go for any shots with a sick baby, as this will completely overpower his immune system; wait until he's completely better. Those who reject any form of immunization claim your child has a stronger immune system without a single jab, especially if you breastfeed exclusively for six months and then continue breastfeeding for at least a year or two, and take a proactive approach to health and nutrition.

'My daughter never had any vaccines or antibiotics. Every bug that goes through her school, she only ever gets the mildest version.'
JANE, MOTHER OF A TEENAGER SHE HAD AT 42

# CHAPTER 11

# *Your Needs*

## THE FOURTH TRIMESTER

*40 Days of Recovery*

In the modern, Western world, once you've given birth and heard the basic instructions on breastfeeding – that's basically it. You're off the conveyer belt to make space for the next pregnant patient. A midwife may come round to answer questions and check you haven't eaten the baby, but no one helps you vacuum, soak all those poo-stained baby grows and whip up healthy meals every 4 hours. Not so in other parts of the world (as you can also see at the end of this chapter), where for around 1 to 3 months new mothers are cared for by family members. The Nepalis, the Turks, the Colombians and many more follow traditions where mum is relieved of all her duties so she can focus on her baby. In China the neighbours traditionally bring energy-boosting and blood-building herbs for the post-partum woman (our neighbours bring plastic toys made in China). The benefit of globalization is that we can pinch other nations' best-kept secrets; *dang gui* (Chinese angelica) has been used for centuries to aid birth recovery and restore the reproductive organs. Take 2 ml of tincture in water three times a day.

---

**AYURVEDIC WISDOM**

In Ayurveda the period after birth is referred to as 'the fourth trimester'. These 3 months are a crucial time for the body of the mother. In ancient Indian philosophy a woman is 'reborn' after she gives birth. It's believed every pore of her body is open, so it's the best time to regenerate and rejuvenate. Because all the channels are open, the body is also vulnerable and blockages are believed to occur more easily. Foods need to be reintroduced slowly because the digestive fire is slower after the mother has given birth. The easiest foods to digest are soups, porridge and semi-solids. The diet of a breastfeeding mother needs to be nutritious because the essence of what she eats goes into her breastmilk. The Gentle Birth Method recommends mothers stay at home for 4 to 6 weeks and rest as much as they can, refrain from household duties and receive Josephson's creative healing and Ayurvedic massage. Traditionally a cloth is tightly bound around the belly from below the breasts all the way down to the pubic joint. This protects and repositions the abdominal organs. It takes approximately 12 months for the uterus to settle back into position, so planning to have children a few years apart is advised. *(Thanks to Dr Seema Datta, Ayurvedic consultant with Gowri Motha, for this information.)*

---

This 40-day resting and regenerating period generally involves mum and progeny staying at home (in Japan women even stay in bed). Apart from mum getting a break, it gives the baby time to adjust to its new environment and stabilize its immune system. In our own history, a lying-in period of a month was routinely observed right up until the 19th century (rest, sleep, silence and solitude). But today we're all in such a rush to get back to work, back to 'normal' and back to our figures. Giving yourself space and time to recover is especially important as a later mother, because not recuperating fully will lead to long-term weaknesses. If you can afford to hire a cleaner, doula or someone to help around the house, do it, do it, do it! (and then send them round to mine, please). A good relationship with your own mother can come in useful, so don't be afraid to become her wanting daughter again (for a limited time, of course). Cooking, cleaning and washing will seem like huge burdens when you're a new mum. So are social commitments, especially those of distant family/psycho neighbours/not-really-a-friend kind. You're likely to be inundated with visitors (bearing gifts, some more useful than others). If you can get the surprise 'drop-ins' to do some housework, fantastic – it might also put them off coming by too often.

## FINDING TIME

A new mum's day is very full because with a baby even *doing nothing* is busy.

Your hours are taken up with feeding, winding, changing nappies, trying to get the baby to sleep, washing more dirty clothes, folding clean clothes and walking around in a daze, otherwise known as exhausted new-mum syndrome. You barely have time to eat, shower or get dressed. The intensity wears off a little after 3 months, and after 6 months you're practically back to normal (this is a blatant lie, but believe it for now). Gone are the sacred days of just *pottering around*. During the precious moments when baby sleeps you will probably charge around at top speed catching up on housework – and there is so much more of it now – rather than *enjoying* this time for yourself. Why relax when you can wipe sticky surfaces, catch up on last month's emails and wash out the inside of the bin? But then don't wonder why you're so exhausted at the end of the day. Fact is – and this won't change for the next

15 years or so – as a mother you *don't* stop and you *don't* get time off unless you actually go away on holiday, without your kids.

> 'I feel like I've regressed to a 1950s housewife now that I've had a baby; the problem is I also have a career – so how do I find space for that? Those 1950s housewives had it much easier.'
>
> **JANE, BABIES AT 39 AND 41**

In the first few weeks, or even months, after birth you could be so high on motherhood that you don't mind your life being turned upside-down. But sooner or later it will be upsetting that you can't complete any tasks. We have endless gadgets invented to save time, but we've become so dependent on them we actually end up with less of it. We've forgotten how to stay still and just pause for a moment. Having a baby forces you to slow down, and it's a great excuse to do less and take some time out. Organization is the key to coping with your new challenges.

## *Small Details*

- Try to make everyday reality enjoyable, rather than being negative about the slog of it.
- Be easy on yourself and a little less perfect, especially when it comes to tidiness.
- Get paid help, if you can afford it.
- Make larger portions when you cook, so you can fill your freezer with healthy, homemade fast-food.
- Juice fruit and veg – it's fast, efficient and so nutritious.
- Do housework with your baby in the sling – babies love the action. Sing while you fold clothes, dust the shelf, etc. because it will cheer you up and soothe the baby.
- Tidy up with your baby, especially when she's a bit older – you can turn it into a game and soon enough she'll copy you (how practical, free labour!).

- Team up with friends who have kids and take turns in minding each other's babies.
- Aim to accomplish only one chore a day – you can't whizz around at your usual pace or you'll drive yourself mad.
- Shop online and get it all delivered to your doorstep.
- Reserve a slot of time each week to do something you can enjoy at your leisure, or arrange weekly treats to look forward to.
- If you commute to work, use that time to read what you want, make lists, sort through documents.
- Fit your baby into your life rather than centring your life around the baby.

## FROM 'ME' TO 'MUM'

You're most likely to be besotted and enamoured with your little cherub. Unless you're Joan Crawford, you'll be focused purely on the survival of your offspring; everything else ceases to exist. This is exactly where the problem lies: you start disappearing.

Don't get me wrong. You may find this *new you* utterly fulfilling, but you're sure to come across moments of frustration and identity crisis – especially being a later mother used to your independence (what do you mean, no more spontaneous coffee breaks?). It's hard putting someone else's needs first (even if it's your mini-me) because it reduces your own flexibility – one of your previously most coveted assets.

To get reconnected to yourself, you have to address your own wants; the Americans have a name for it: *self-care*. We women are complex emotionally and hormonally – hence our mystery and beauty – and we have to respect this before anyone else will. Becoming a mother will turn your identity on its head, and then when it does finally veer back it exposes you in a new, different light. Give yourself time to adjust and don't feel guilty about taking time for yourself. It took me a good year – maybe even two – to feel vaguely like myself again. Well, myself as a mother, that is.

## Back to Me

- Go for long walks – by yourself – don't talk to anyone and try not to think too much. Relax, stop worrying, clear your mind, soak up nature and breathe.

- Meet a girlfriend for lunch – the one who reminds you of all the fun, crazy things you did and what a cool/bright/brave woman you were – and still are.

- Attend yoga classes at least once a week, religiously like mass.

- Have a long bath and pamper yourself like a queen.

- Do something brain-stimulating and cultural: visit an exhibition you thought you'd miss or a museum you've always wanted to see properly. Indulge in your time alone, feeling settled and safe that you're a mum now.

- Think of all the incredible things you've done, the amazing adventures you've been on, the wild times you've enjoyed and feel grateful for them. Realize that you were ready to move on to the next step in adulthood. Feel lucky that it all worked out and you were able to experience becoming a mother.

- Go dancing. Take a course in something exotic you always wanted to learn; any dancing is good but especially belly dancing connects you to your centre.

- Make a shrine for the new you. Arrange some flowers on a table; add a picture, card, or anything pretty you like. Make wishes for yourself.

- When your little one is a bit bigger and can cope without you, go away – by yourself – for the night, weekend or even a week. You will need to keep pinching yourself. You'll miss your baby terribly but she will survive just fine without you.

There will also be moments when you feel your strength and independence returning.

- Be patient. In a couple of years your child will be gone for hours and you'll be left with yourself to contend with and lots of time on your hands.

NB All of the above means you have to get your partner/mother/best friend/sitter to look after the baby – that is the whole point!

## FATIGUE

### *Foggy-headed*

Not letting someone sleep is a known form of torture, so when you are woken five times a night and then forced to get up at 7 a.m., it can feel a tad on the rough side. Many new mums say lack of sleep is the hardest aspect of motherhood, and it rubs off on everything else: you become moody, irritable and your other problems massively exaggerated. According to one survey, 8 out of 10 mothers say lack of sleep puts their relationship under 'immense strain', and 81 per cent say it causes rows.[1]

However – and please repeat this to yourself every time you feel exhausted – THIS IS A SHORT, INTENSE PERIOD OF YOUR LIFE THAT WILL PASS, faster than you think (before you know it your child will be asking for a tattoo). Those early, sleep-dazed months are also deliciously intimate. I still remember looking into my baby's dreamy eyes when only we two were awake in the world. His gentle sighs of contentment as he fell asleep after a feed and woke up with a smile to the dawn chorus were precious moments that went so fast.

If you're having a particularly bad day – after a particularly interrupted night – I wouldn't attempt cutting vegetables with a sharp knife, filling in your tax form, learning macramé or even driving. Studies reveal that sleep deprivation can make you drive worse than if you were drunk at the wheel. Plus you probably have a baby screaming blue murder in the back. Show me a mother who doesn't fret and turn around to check her child and I'll show you a hormonal young man who test-drives a sports car slowly without revving the engine.

## LIGHT RELIEF

I know plenty of later mums who complain their energy levels aren't the same as when they studied all night for A levels and went to 24-hour raves (sometimes in the same weekend), or that they have extra wrinkles because they didn't get those 8.5 hours of beauty kip. The main thing that'll help you recuperate from those broken nights is that wonderful Latin invention: *La Siesta*. If there's one thing I learned living in Spain, it's how these boisterous folk manage to keep going. They leave the house at 10 p.m., snack on tapas at 11, chase their kids across the plaça at midnight (wonder what Gina Ford would say to that?) and then slowly wander home around 1 a.m. – and that's only those who don't get drunk and go dancing from 3 a.m. until dawn. The secret to this is having a kip in the middle of the day. From 3 p.m. until around 5 p.m., all the Iberians (expect those doing business with banks abroad) go to see Nod. Woe betide anyone who dares phone during those sacred hours of snooze.

### *How to Feel Rested without a Good Night's Sleep*

- Cat-nap during the day with your baby.
- If you can't cat-nap (a paid job, perhaps?) then close your eyes while you commute, blocking out any additional stress by listening to music.

- Do a vigorous 15-minute yoga session with a 2-minute meditation at the end.
- Go for a brisk walk.
- Take an omega 3 supplement daily.
- Float in salt water (but, as most of us don't live next to a warm sea, take a bath with salts instead).
- Stay well hydrated, snack on nuts and eat regular meals.
- Go to bed stupidly early, like 9 p.m., at least twice a week.
- Check your nutrient levels: maybe you have a potassium weakness or thyroid deficiency.
- Avoid processed foods and too much sugar – drinking more coffee and eating more chocolate may be immediate pick-me-ups, but you feel worse after the buzz wears off and they drain your reserves.
- If you're seriously going mad, hire a night nanny or get someone to look after your baby during the day so you can sleep.
- If you're bottle-feeding or expressing breastmilk you could ask your partner if he'll kindly take over a few nightshifts. I just loved it when Tony Blair said he got up in the night to change Leo's nappies, despite having a country to run. Now if a prime minister can do it, so can your lazy bones (or maybe it's time he got better at PR to convince you he's 'sharing responsibilities'). Yes, you will fight over who gets more sleep, and you may decide to get divorced once a week. But like I said, *this phase passes* and soon you'll be sleeping like a baby again (how on earth did that expression sneak in there?).

## The 'I'm Not Tired, I Just Haven't Slept for 5 Months' Test

You know you're sleep deprived when:
- you leave the phone in the fridge

- you throw dirty laundry into the toilet
- you use your lipstick as eyeshadow
- you day-dream about duvets
- you feel like you've just come down off acid (just imagine!)
- you put nappies on the outside of your baby's jeans
- you can't get past the first 30 seconds of Later with Jools Holland
- you walk past people you know on the street but always notice how dirty the kerb is
- you leave the shopping on the roof of the car and drive off
- your vision blurs even with glasses
- when your partner suggests sex you think it's the most hilarious thing he's ever said, turn over and snore immediately.

## FEELING BLUE

*Why So Sad?*

Adjusting to motherhood takes time. There's a period of upheaval and transition until you get used to your new life. Practically all women have deeply melancholic moments, days or even weeks after birth. Feelings of failure, resentment and an unexplained sadness are all normal; 10 to 20 per cent of new mothers get seriously depressed.

Postnatal depression (PND) is allegedly hormonally driven; some experts believe it's due to a sharp drop in progesterone, while others believe it's a sudden lack of the mood-elevator oestrogen. However, not just hormones are to blame for making millions of bouncy new mums weepy – there are other culprits.

The massive responsibility of doing this baby thing practically alone in the isolation of your own home is daunting. Since we ventured away from tribal villages into our little houses where we can lock the door and other people out, we've become increasingly more miserable (and the richer and more isolated we become, the more depressed we get, as Oliver James proved brilliantly in his book *Affluenza*). As the famous saying, 'It takes a village to raise a child' suggests, in an ideal world a new mum is fully integrated into the community and other members chip in to look after the baby – for free, it has to be said.

Depression is also linked to fatigue, with tests showing that even adoptive parents suffer from a version of PND related to lack of sleep. Other contributing factors to PND are lack of postnatal care, education level, single household status and less clear-cut reasons such as crisis in identity – something which new mothers are particularly vulnerable to. I don't know a single woman out of all my fab friends who didn't have a little crumbling of self-esteem after birth, often to do with insensitive comments by partners such as, 'Have you looked at yourself in the mirror lately?' – but more to that Mount Everest of a gripe later.

The good news is that various studies show later mothers suffer less from PND. An Australian study found the reason to be that later mothers are more mature and resilient, due to greater life experience. They are shown to be more adaptive at coping with challenges. The older mothers who did suffer from PND were more than twice as likely to seek help than the younger ones.[2]

## PND *Alert*

You're constantly exhausted, you feel empty, you can't concentrate, you feel guilty about not being a good mother, you might even have thoughts of harming your baby (morbid thoughts are apparently a typical symptom of PND). You may also find yourself in tears at any time of the day for reasons you can't explain. Insomnia, lack of appetite, panic attacks and compulsive behaviour are signs of PND.

## Happier Bunny

First of all, make sure you're not run-down due to inadequate diet (if it's not clear by now, go ahead and stick that packet lasagne in the microwave). There are simple measures to reduce the flow of stress hormones, such as getting out of the house to meet a friend, taking a walk, practising positive visualizations or having a soak in the bath. Use some essential oils to lift your mood such as geranium, neroli or rose. Also try exercising regularly, because this will release endorphins which make you feel better. Meet people who cheer you up, not ones who make you moan more or who have similar problems to you (this may mean avoiding new-mum groups sometimes) and do things that add some joy to your life to boost your love hormones. Oxytocin and prolactin flow naturally during pregnancy and birth and continue to increase if you're breastfeeding, so keep feeding and make frequent eye contact with your baby. If you can manage a little smile now and again, it will lift your spirits as well as hers.

If subtle changes aren't making a difference, book some massages, bodywork, cranial osteopathy or other complementary treatments. Speak to a counsellor or try Cognitive Behavioural Therapy (CBT), which works well on mild to moderate depression.

Feeling down could be related to old issues from your past cropping up, even as far back as your own infancy. A technique called *metamorphic healing* has been shown to release tension accumulated during your own time in the womb and early childhood. In becoming a mother, it's possible that you have triggered some painful cellular memory. Rather than blaming yourself for being a bad mother, use this opportunity to work on raising your own awareness. Children can be the world's best catalysts for self-discovery and healing processes.

'I got very depressed after my son was born – I had so much to do and so many expectations. Eventually I went for hypnotherapy and found out my own birth was very traumatic. I went to speak to my mother who said when she came home from the hospital with me, she found my father – an alcoholic womanizer – having sex with another woman. My mother panicked and tried to strangle me. As she told me this I could feel the pain and trauma in my body. I went back to the therapist and it's like we put the puzzle together. With this information I was released and was able to forgive myself for being depressed.'

**NINA, SECOND BABY AT 35**

If you're suffering badly from PND you'll probably avoid bonding deeply with your baby which can be harmful in the long run. A psychotherapist can help to improve interaction between the both of you. The therapist may point out deficits but also give you useful resources. You'll be shown examples of how to tackle simple, everyday tasks such as cooking and shopping with the baby, which seem impossible if you're depressed. You don't have to be perfect, a good enough mother is all your baby needs.

## Getting Back into Shape

Some women are models and film stars with personal trainers and privates chefs; these ladies always look skinny posing with newborns, but most of us mortals of the female species need to be more patient. You do get your body back, including a flat-ish stomach – it just doesn't happen within minutes of giving birth. Remember, it took you 9 months to get that big, so it will take at least 6 to 9 months to get trim again. If you're breastfeeding the pounds might just drop off you, or quite the opposite can happen – some women get so hungry breastfeeding they actually put on weight. You shouldn't diet when you're nursing but you can cut down on fast food, fatty foods, sugar and high-carb snacks such as crisps and cakes; replace with big salads and healthy smoothies for the sweet kick. If you need to look good for a special occasion (shot-gun post-partum wedding, maybe?) there are some great tricks, such as wearing a type of cycling short under your clothes. This corset for the yum mum comes in a wide array of crowd-pleasing colours, shapes and styles.

Whatever your current out-of-shapeness, a bit of exercise will make you feel better and more energetic. In the first weeks and months I only felt like exercising gently: walking in the fresh air and a bit of yoga. Yoga and Pilates are really effective because you can target the most worn-out areas. Rebuilding your pelvic floor is essential if you want to avoid wetting yourself every time you sneeze/laugh/cough/can't make it to the loo in time. If you're lucky enough to live in a forward-thinking neighbourhood you're likely to have access to 'Baby and Me' yoga classes. These can be lots of fun, relaxing and bonding, even if not necessarily a sweaty workout. Some mothers resort to sticking on a DVD and 'Ohming' in the front room. Anything you can fit into your schedule is basically a bonus.

If you have stubborn weight to shift, then a more radical approach is called for – that is, the treadmill treatment. Cardio exercise gets your metabolism going and burns off excess fat. Once you've recovered from birth (like 6 months later) and feel ready to attack the pounds, go running, cycling, spinning, swimming, sweaty dancing (or how about sweaty sex?) and do it for at least 45 minutes (you might have to hire a stud for the latter option, as most new dads are pathetic at anything over 7 minutes). I always marvel at the svelte mums in New York's parks as they run laps with their babies in those pneumatic jogging prams. If all else fails, go to India for a few weeks – it works for me every time.

# CAREER CALLS

## *Work-life Balance*

By the time you've got into the swing of your new baby-rules lifestyle, it's usually time to go back to that other thing you did before mini-Kaiser came along. For every mother who can't get enough of all that scone-baking, finger-painting fun, there's the mother who's desperate to get back to the office to chat about non-poop-related matters, drink a coffee before it gets cold and finish a task without being interrupted. Most of us would like a bit of both: the perfect work-life balance, money and sanity with plenty of free time. According to my *Right Time Baby* survey, later mothers have more flexibility when it comes to returning to work, thanks to having clocked up enough mileage in the careers department, *and* some life savings. Many use the transition of motherhood to go freelance, downshift, start a business or 'portfolio career' or take a well-deserved sabbatical.

Going back to work on a part-time or job-sharing basis is an option many are able to negotiate (the advantages of being older than your boss), as well as working from home a few days a week. I know a dozen or so women who work while their partners are stay-at-home dads. You bet these dads have the typical 'housewife' complaints of frustration, lack of confidence and being taken for granted – but guess who gets really jealous and still ends up washing up after dinner?

Stay-at-home mums (and dads) are a 20th-century invention of Western society. Mothers have gone out to work, with their babies strapped to them or cared for by other family members, since the dawn of time. Historically in our society the upper classes didn't need to toil and labour but they had nurses to look after their kids, so they were hardly hands-on mums, either. In our parents' generation the perfect middle-class mother gave up her job, nurtured her kids, excelled in the kitchen and even managed to do her hair before hubby came home. Today, most of us have jobs as well as trying to be good mothers. Aiming to fulfil both roles means we push ourselves to the limit and face enormous guilt for any shortcomings. Leaving your child crying with someone else while you run off to work is not a pleasant way to start the day. However, the key to happiness is to ditch the guilt, get on with it and thrive. You're *having it all*, isn't that what you always wanted?

## Who Cares for Precious?

Childcare options have improved vastly over the last decade, but they're still costly and you need impeccable organizational skills to work around them. The easiest and cheapest option is getting someone from the family to care for your child. It does make it harder to impose the 'no sugar, no TV, no sleeping with the gerbil' rules because without a salary you're not the boss. But it does mean your child can spend the day in familiar surroundings with someone who will love them nearly as much as you do. The other more expensive 'in-the-home' option is hiring a nanny or au pair. It's worth choosing very carefully and really checking those references. You want a great nanny with glowing recommendations (call previous employers!), not one who eats all your ice-cream, runs up your phone bill and snogs boys (or, dare we even go there: your husband) on the couch. Childminders are cheaper because they usually have more children to look after in their own house. If you're choosing a nursery, go on recommendations and check the Ofsted reports; smaller nurseries with a low staff turnover are preferable. Children over 2 often do well in a nursery environment, but the general consensus is that not many nurseries have the ideal set-up for small babies.

With all the childcare options, it's worth slowly getting your child used to its new carer(s) and building up the time you spend away. You need a back-up plan if your child is sick; can you take time off work, or will a family member take over? You also need a good routine in order to get out of the house on time.

The pressure will be on to spend quality time with junior outside of working hours. Some mothers say they enjoy their children more when they're not around them all day. It's a good idea to focus solely on your infant when you reunite, even if you're stressed because you've spent hours in front of a computer and now have to get the dinner ready. If you're feeling confused, tired or guilty this will be transmitted to your child, so try to stay calm and then off-load on your husband when the baby's tucked up in bed. Or perhaps not.

## RELATIONSHIPS

### *Where Did the Love Go?*

Relationships can change quite dramatically when you have a first child (and become even more strained after a second or third). As wanted as it may be, a first baby is a demanding third addition to a previously absorbed-with-each-other twosome. It's the end of one relationship and the start of a new one, with more people involved. Your focus will shift onto the baby, showering it with attention, affection, kisses and cuddles – rather than each other. What's most shocking is how old-fashioned gender roles suddenly appear. This is particularly hard for us daughters of the bra-burners to stomach; we're so used to our independence, own money and freedom. Asking a man for favours or cash is probably something you've fought against all your life. New mothers often feel trapped and unsupported, whereas fathers feel left out and pressurized to be the breadwinner. You start complaining about how hard everything is and he displays passive-aggressive behaviour and labels you a nag (and don't we all just love being called that?). Before you know it he comes out with patriarchal comments you'd never have expected like: 'Why did you have to spend so much on this?', 'But you can't be tired, you've been at home all day,' 'Couldn't you at least have managed to get dinner ready?'

An unmarried friend I interviewed has the following advice:

'It's not very romantic but I would negotiate beforehand issues such as money, insurance, housework and time off from the baby. If you're giving up your career for a while you need to know he's supporting you, and that includes the money missing from your pension. You need time for yourself at least once or twice a week and this is a great opportunity for him to see how hard it can be looking after an infant. In Berlin it's become part of the culture: on Sunday mornings the city's full of dads with kids, even the cafés have installed special *happy hours* for them.'

MECHTHILD, BABY AT 43

Parenting is the lowest paid, least valued activity in society. Most women crave some appreciation for what they're doing – at least from their partners – and less criticism. This goes both ways, of course: he criticizes you for being overanxious about the baby, and you criticize him for running off to the pub. My partner's sarcastic comment: 'She used to be fun, now she's a typical mother' (nice, eh?) says it all. We never intend to morph into our own mothers, but shouldering most of the responsibility for the baby just does that to you – at least for a while.

One thing you can do, apart from getting a lobotomy, is to really allow your partner to share (not just look after or help with) the baby. Children need their fathers' input. A study at Lancaster University showed that where fathers were involved with baby care, mothers found breastfeeding easier, children performed better at exams and were less likely to have a criminal record by age 21. So tell Dad to get with it now if he wants to avoid visiting junior in prison. Involving him as much as possible ensures he feels needed – that is, less useless. It also means he's as knackered as you are and thus has less energy to throw strops. A mistake many mothers make is interfering (I'm so guilty of it). Best let him do it his way! If this means the baby's wearing odd socks and a cardigan covered in sick, so be it. Get out of the house – *what you don't see won't upset you* – and book yourself in for a haircut or other treat (yes, these necessities will be known as 'treats' from now on). If the baby cries non-stop in his company, you can try wearing his shirt before he does, so it smells of you. Repeat the mantra, 'I let go in the face of chaos. I let go completely.'

Aside from having more things to fight about (and this is before religion, discipline or schooling are even mentioned!) the other big adjustment is having less time for each other. So often you end up as cohabiting childminders, rugby-passing the baby in the hallway, exchanging information on whether it has pooped, fed and slept before running off to your other commitments. You need to reconnect, which means *spending time together alone* – without dribbler.

The UK-based charity Relate says new parents should go on a date with each other once a week. Trying to achieve that is as realistic as expecting Brad Pitt to walk through the door when you call a plumber (sorry plumbers, admittedly some of you are quite handsome). Even if you manage to go out, it won't be the same as before. If you can avoid talking just about the baby, then a whole range of other things may spoil your evening such as:

- You end up fighting. This can be about anything as minor as him not using his knife to more important things like why his mother should stick her nose out of your child's upbringing.
- His eyes glaze over because he's not as into the pros and cons of baby-led weaning as you are.
- Your eyes glaze over because football scores and office politics seem banal in the face of your tasks.

- The fact that you're boring each other makes you wonder whether you've grown apart (and the inevitable next step is filing for divorce?)
- You're too exhausted to enjoy the evening.
- You'll definitely be too exhausted to have sex when you get home.
- You're not drinking alcohol (to avoid gin in the breastmilk) so his jokes are flat.
- You both agree it's better to stay in and watch telly next time.

Despite all the above-mentioned hiccups, relationships do massively benefit from communal offspring. Shared love for a child will fuse you together forever. Part of yourself and the love of your life (well, until recently!) came out as the cutest little parcel, so something about your coupling must be all right.

In ancient Tantric philosophy it's believed we are all divine beings, so this means recognizing divinity in your other half. Or quite simply, respect and honour each other. Appreciate what he does and he'll appreciate you. Say thanks, look into each other's eyes and touch regularly. Just sharing a hug can make such a big difference.

## Parents Don't Have Sex

Yes, I know this is the probably the last thing on your mind right now. Let it stay there, I'm definitely not going to rush you back into this one. I would even say, lie to your partner about how long the doctor said you should wait. What's 3, 4, even 6 months in the face of aching pains and constant fatigue? Your life is sensually supersaturated with an infant, and there comes a point when you just want to be *in your own space* without being licked, sucked and needed. If you're breastfeeding this is even more of the case – our mammalian cousins are not receptive to the male when they're lactating, and in many societies breastfeeding women don't bonk. Also, physically you're a little 'dried up' down there, due to all those essential body juices being used to make milk. This is only for the first months, so if you're breastfeeding for the long term, don't worry, you *will* get your mojo back before the menopause. I really hope you have an understanding, family-orientated partner who doesn't run off with 'Mary from the office' until you resurface. If all else fails send him kinky text messages promising him a raunchy night (at, say, the next lunar eclipse).

It's not just you who went through transition alley. Your lover became a father. Some women may find this new incarnation even more appealing, but the reality is he'll also have bags under his eyes big enough for the weekly shopping. Lack of sleep spoils a couple's love-life because, given the chance to lie horizontal, most prefer sleep to more activity.

It's a known fact that even though love needs emotional closeness, eroticism likes distance, freedom and adventure. Being parents with a dependant is probably the least reckless you can get. How can you desire what you already have? This is where we go one level deeper – lift to basement, watch out for the 'mummies' in the dark – and find something richer and much more meaningful. Lovemaking once you have a child is really that: through your making love, life was created. Keep it flowing!

## SINGLE AND MUM

Many women with increasing age decide to have a baby on their own if the right partner doesn't show up. The obvious disadvantages of single motherhood are limited time, money and resources. It can also be lonely. The big advantages are that you have more time to yourself (when the baby sleeps) and you're much freer to do as you please. You don't have to schedule a board meeting to discuss whether to feed your child pasta or brown rice for dinner, whether you should cut his hair or which school to send him to. You don't have to negotiate anything. All the single mums I know have an extremely close bond with their offspring. It's far better for a child to be in harmonious relationship with its mother than living with an example of how dysfunctional a relationship can possibly be. Ancient civilizations and cultures worshipped mother goddesses who weren't attached to male partners and many indigenous, matriarchal societies don't recognize fatherhood.

## Becoming a Family

Once you've had a baby, you're the mother of your mother-in-law's grandchild. Get it? Your child is linked to *that* woman by blood – it's her baby's baby. Your genes have been pooled together via munchkin. And all those 'outlaws' and other extensions of your partner are also related to your little precious. So, however much you'd rather pretend it's just your side of the family that counts, you're going to have to put up with them, at least occasionally. They may love your child more than they'll ever love you, but if that means they're fantastic babysitters, who cares? They may even be able to weekend-sit, so you can go to 'honeymoon bliss' with your man and see if a little brother or sister wants to join your happy family. Oh boy, are you sure? You want the whole game to start all over again?

## ALL AROUND THE WORLD

Just because we carry babies around in car seats and pacify them with rubber teats doesn't mean everyone thinks that's such a great idea. Here are some different customs from around the globe.

*Aborigines:* Traditionally believe a spirit-child selects his parents before entering a woman's body around the time of conception.

The father makes first contact with the spirit-child through a dream, sometimes even years before the child is born. The aborigines believe the main cause of pregnancy is the father's pre-conception dream, rather than sex. Sometimes he passes the spirit over to his wife in a second dream or carries it in his hair and places it near her navel. The spirit-child is believed to be more ancient than, and completely independent of, any living person.

*Bali:* Newborns are believed to be the incarnation of a released ancestor. For the first 42 days mother and baby are thought to be in a state of spiritual impurity. At the end of this period a ritual is performed, offerings are made and all the vices that accompanied the child into birth are asked to depart. The newborn's feet are not allowed to touch the earth for 210 days after birth.

*China:* Pregnant women are encouraged to think only peaceful, calming thoughts because of the ancient belief that what you think affects your heart and the unborn child. A pregnant woman is also forbidden to attend funerals as these might attract evil spirits.

*Colombia:* Mothers rest for 40 days after birth to recover their bodies. They are not to exert any effort or travel. Another family member is expected to take over the daily chores.

*Congo:* Mothers regularly sing their babies in-utero the same song so they'll remember it after birth.

*Hindu:* High-caste children are breastfed up to three to five years by their mothers. During this time the fathers, traditionally Brahman priests, spend most of their time in deep meditation.

*India:* The entire community works to make pregnant women feel as happy and peaceful as possible. This is because pregnant women are believed to have a direct link to their babies. At the time of birth an opening ritual takes place. Women let their hair down, remove all jewellery and open anything that can be closed, including the doors of their house. It's traditionally thought that by breastfeeding, mothers give their children their characteristics.

*Java:* They say the womb is like a cave where the baby sits like a mystic meditating and preparing for his life on earth.

*Japan:* Custom dictates that mothers stay in bed with their newborns for 21 days. They eat special seaweed to stimulate milk production.

*Mali:* The placenta is washed, dried, put in a basket and buried by the father. It's thought that the placenta has a supernatural link to the baby and can affect his mood. A proverb says that if you don't breastfeed, your child won't recognize you.

*Maoris:* Traditionally believe that pregnant women should be protected and guarded with respect. Gestating women need to be relaxed and comfortable because the baby is fully aware of what's going on in its environment. Fathers are taught to perform *Haputanga*, a form of belly massage, body alignment and acupressure, to ease pregnancy discomforts and facilitate birth. After birth the mother's internal organs are repositioned and her body is realigned through *Haputanga*. The baby is given cranial-sacral therapy to remove birth trauma, sleep problems, colic and depression.

*Malaysia:* Mothers are given hot baths infused with fragrant leaves to restore 'heat', health and balance. A paste of garlic, ginger, tamarind and lime is rubbed on her belly to help the uterus shrink. She is then given a body massage, including her breasts for improved milk flow.

*Pygmies:* Carry babies for the first year in skin-to-skin contact. If clothing is needed it's wrapped around both, never between them. During the first year the baby is never separated from the mother, although the father also plays with, hugs and holds the baby as much as the mother. Babies are nursed for five years and rarely cry. Breasts are considered sacred and reserved for the child.

*Quiché of Guatemala:* Have a ceremony when the mother is 7 months pregnant where she tells her child in a loud voice all about the forests, mountains, rivers and the surroundings into which it will soon be born. This is a way of welcoming the baby and preparing it for its future life on earth.

*Taiwan:* Labouring mothers are expected to control their emotions and not to cry out during birth. As Buddhists they believe that suffering in childbirth is linked to sins the mother committed in a previous life.

# *Afterword*

Never before has change been as accelerated as it is today; time is literally speeding up. Many scientists, astrologers, mystics and leading thinkers agree that we will experience a kind of rebirth or shift as the planet comes to the end of a 5,000-year cycle (and the beginning of the next). For the first time in modern history, science and religion are coming together. Western rationale and eastern spirituality are converging. It's believed we're entering an age where feminine strengths will be integrated with the powerful masculine mind that has ruled the planet for the past 2,000 years. An important new world view is that life for humans on the planet has a collective, cosmic aim beyond individual endeavour. We're moving from the 'me' to the 'we', from the ego to connecting with our higher selves and the Divine. We're basically moving into our hearts. Cutting-edge research in neurocardiology shows that the heart contains neural structures, or brain cells. It is even believed that integrating this 'fourth brain' is the next evolutionary step for us as human beings. By waking up to a new, greater form of intelligence and becoming more conscious, we may find a way to live in harmony with the resources of Mother Earth, rather than dominating, exploiting and destroying her. Our plants, animals, oceans, rivers and soils are bearing the burden of the impact of human activity and waste. We ourselves are suffering as fertility declines and babies are born with toxic chemicals and industrial pollutants in the blood of their umbilical cords. It's time to show up and be more authentic and truthful. A pregnant woman nurtures the next generation – future consciousness – in her womb. We should never underestimate the importance of that role or the privilege of protecting this precious seed of full human potential.

We are never as connected to *what this is all about* as when we're pregnant, giving birth and caring for a newborn. It really is our moment of truth.

Modern science is finally proving what our ancient ancestors intuitively knew about conception, pregnancy, birth and babies. They were in touch with their divine selves and they respected Mother Earth. We've lived though centuries of systems and rules that interfered with basic rites. We've come to a point where we don't even know our own bodies or instincts any more. I believe that in order to go forward we have to look right back to our origins and see how it fits with what we know today. This begins by simply acknowledging our true mammalian nature and seeing who we really are – essentially spiritual beings governed by love.

Motherhood is physically and emotionally demanding, but it is above all a spiritual journey. Having children is an immense gift because it means we have the chance to rediscover real love; the love that connects us with each other. A child shows you places within that you didn't know or you forgot existed. You get to relive everything through untainted, wondering eyes. Becoming a parent is also a unique opportunity to raise your awareness. If you're suddenly a role model you may start looking more carefully at your own behaviour. Often your child is your teacher; especially many of the more spiritually attuned children being born today. If we can be open to what our children have to show us, we can grow through them and genuinely become *better* human beings. We influence our children and our children influence us. It's all interconnected, as we fulfil our individual and collective destiny, in remembering who we really are.

# *References*

## CHAPTER ONE

1. Mirowsky, J., 'Age at first birth, health and mortality', *Journal of Health and Social Behavior* 46 (2005): 32–50; see also Mirowsky, John quoted in *Psychology Today* (October 11ᵗʰ 2008)
2. Viau, Paula A., 'An exploration of health concerns and health promotion behaviours in pregnant women over age 35', *The American Journal of Maternal/Child Nursing* 27 (2002): 328–34
3. Grusso, Pietro, 'La Maternita dopo 35 anni', *Richerche di Psicologia* 25 (2002): 39–55
4. Hills-Bonczyk, S. G. *et al.*, 'Women's experiences with breastfeeding longer than 12 months', *Birth* 21 (1994): 206–12; and *The Right Time* baby survey showed 8 per cent of later mothers didn't breastfeed, 49 per cent breastfed more than 6 months, 24 per cent over 12 months
5. Mirowsky, J. and Ross, C., 'Depression, parenthood and age at first birth', *Social Science and Medicine* (2001): 1–18
6. Gregory, Elizabeth, *Ready: Why Women Are Embracing the New Later Motherhood* (Basic Books, 2008)
7. Ibid.
8. 'Worried about being a late mum?', *The Observer* (28ᵗʰ October 2007) quoting study published in *Journal of Epidemiology and Community Health*
9. Various studies all confirm older mothers live longer: The New England Centenarian Study, Boston University Medical Centre; Mirowsky, J., Population Research Centre, University of Texas; Smith K., University of Utah; Helle S., University of Turku, Finland

10. Gregory, Elizabeth, op. cit.

11. Mirowsky, John, quoted in *Psychology Today* (October 11th 2008) and *The Observer* (28th October 2007)

12. Steiner, A. Z. and Paulson, R. J., 'Motherhood after age 50: an evaluation of parenting stress and physical functioning', *Fertil Steril* 87 (2007): 1327–32

13. Langer, Ellen, *Counterclockwise* (Hodder, 2010); *Mindfulness* (Westview Press, 1990)

14. Austad, Steve, *Why We Age* (John Wiley & Sons, 1999)

15. *The Daily Telegraph* (22nd July 2010) and Gillespie, D. O. *et al.*, 'Pair-bonding modifies the age-specific intensities of natural selection on human female fecundity', *American Naturalist* 176 (2010): 159–69

16. Tanaka, Sakiko, 'Parental leave and child health across OECD Countries', *Economic Journal,* February 2005

17. As calculated by the *Liverpool Victoria Friendly Society*

18. Schwartz, Pepper, *Peer Marriage* (Simon & Schuster, 1994)

19. Oxford University study by Sullivan, Oriel cited in *The Telegraph* (April 7th, 2010)

## CHAPTER TWO

1. Dobbyn, Sarah, *The Fertility Diet* (Simon & Schuster, 2008); West, Zita, *Zita West's Guide to Getting Pregnant* (Harper Thorsons, 2005); Glenville, Marilyn, *Getting Pregnant – Faster* (Kyle Cathie, 2008); also see QualityLowInputFood – a £12 million, four-year EU study: http://www.qlif.org/

2. Carlson, E., *et al.*, 'Semen quality among members of organic food associations in Zeeland, Denmark', *Lancet* 347 (1996): 1844; Dobbyn, Sarah, op. cit.: 106

3. Abell, A., *et al.*, 'High sperm density among members of the Organic Farmers' Association', *Lancet* 343 (1995): 1498

4.  Study conducted by Dr Gabriel Cousens at the *Tree of Life Rejuvenation Centre* in Arizona in 2005. See also Dobbyn, Sarah, op. cit.: 173

5.  Pizzi, William, Barnhart, June, *et al.*, *Neurobehavioral Toxicology* 2 (1979): 1–4. See also Cannon, Emma *The Baby-Making Bible* (Rodale, 2010): 63; Dooley, Michael, *Fit for Fertility* ( Hodder, 2007): 101; West, Zita op. cit.: 94

6.  Chavarro, Jorge and Willett, Walter C., *The Fertility Diet* (McGraw-Hill, 2007): This book brings together research from the eight-year *Nurses' Health Study* involving 18,555 women aged between 24 and 42

7.  Dobbyn, Sarah op. cit.: 41–42

8.  Cannon, Emma op. cit.: 65; Dooley, Michael op. cit.: 101; West, Zita op. cit.: 94

9.  Chavarro and Willett, op. cit.

10. Cannon, Emma op. cit.: 44–45

11. Dobbyn, Sarah op. cit.: 204–206

12. Chunyuan, F., McLaughlin, J.K, *et al.*, 'Maternal levels of perfluorinated chemicals and subfecundity', *Human Reproduction* 24.5 (2009): 1200–1205

13. Information sheet published by UK charity Foresight

14. Cannon, Emma op. cit. and West, Zita op. cit.: 174

15. Curtis K. M., Savitz, D. A. *et al.*, 'Effects of cigarette smoking, caffeine consumption, and alcohol intake on fecundability,' *American Journal of Epidemiology* 146 (1997): 32–41

16. Chavarro and Willett, op. cit.

17. Dobbyn, Sarah op. cit.: 69

18. Dobbyn, Sarah, op. cit.: 72

19. 'Study links stress to infertility' on *www.naturalnews.com* (September 6th 2006)

20. Carlsen, E., *et al.*, 'Evidence for the decreasing quality of

semen during the past 50 years', *British Medical Journal* 305 (1992): 609–13

21. 'Out for the Count' in *The Independent* (26ᵗʰ April 2010)

# CHAPTER THREE

1. *The British Medical Journal* (February 2008) collated results from seven separate trials conducted in Western countries with 1366 women. Acupuncture during IVF showed to increase the chances of pregnancy by 67 per cent, an increase in continuing pregnancy by 87 per cent and a 91 per cent increase in live births

2. UK charity Foresight, '1990–1993 study of preconceptual care and pregnancy outcome', *Journal of Nutritional and Environmental Medicine* 5 (1995): 205–208

3. Kang Zou, Zhe Yuan *et al.*, 'Producing of offspring from a germline stem cell line derived from neonatal ovaries', *Nature Cell Biology* 11 (2009): 631–36

4. Lane Wong L., Legro, R., 'Efficacy of oocytes donated by older women in an oocyte donation programme', *Human Reproduction* 11.4 (1996): 820–23

5. Bhattacharya, S., Harrild, K., *et al.*, 'Clomifene citrate or unstimulated intrauterine insemination compared with expectant management for unexplained infertility: pragmatic randomised controlled trial', *British Medical Journal* 337 (2008): 716

6. Aughagen-Stephanos, Ute, *Damit mein Baby Bleibt* (Kösel Verlag, 2009): 43

7. Kneale, D., Joshi, H., 'Postponement and Childlessness', *Demographic Research* 19.58 (2008): 1935–68; see also *Institute for Public Policy Research* (IPPR)

## CHAPTER FOUR

1. Scher, Jonathan and Dix, Carol *Preventing Miscarriage* (HarperCollins, 2005): 30
2. Regan, Lesley and Rai, Raj, 'Recurrent Miscarriage', *Lancet* 368 (2006): 601–11
3. Ibid.
4. Scher and Dix op. cit.: 9 and Rousselot, Susan, *Avoiding Miscarriage* (Sea Change Press, 2007): 17
5. Peppone, L., *et al.*, 'Associations between adult and childhood secondhand smoke exposures and fecundity and fetal loss among women who visited a cancer hospital', *Tobacco Control* 18 (2009): 115–20; Venners, S., *et al.*, 'Paternal Smoking and Pregnancy Loss', *American Journal of Epidemiology* 159.10 (2004): 993–1001
6. Kesmodel, U., 'Moderate alcohol intake in pregnancy and the risk of spontaneous abortion', *Alcohol and Alcholism* 37.1 (2002): 87–92
7. Infante-Rivard, C., *et al.*, 'Fetal loss associated with caffeine intake before and during pregnancy', *Journal of the American Medical Association* 270.24 (1993): 2940–43
8. Rousselot, Susan op. cit.: 47

## CHAPTER FIVE

1. Foetal development taken from various sources including Murkoff, Heidi and Mazel, Sharon, *What to Expect When You're Expecting* (Simon & Schuster, 2008); Bellybutton, *Das Grosse Schwangerschaftsbuch* (Wunderlich, 2006); websites such as babycentre.co.uk and swissmom.ch
2. Oren, D.A., *et al.*, 'An open trial of morning light therapy for treatment of antepartum depression', *American Journal of Psychiatry* 159.4 (2002): 666–69

3. Staples, J., et al., 'Low maternal exposure to ultraviolet radiation in pregnancy, month of birth, and risk of multiple sclerosis in offspring: longitudinal study', *British Medical Journal* 340 (2010): 1640

4. Sayers A., et al., 'Estimated maternal ultraviolet B exposure levels in pregnancy influence skeletal development of the child', *Journal of Clinical Endocrinology and Metabolism* 94.3 (2009): 765-71

5. Murphy, Michael et al., *The Physical and Psychological Effects of Meditation* (Institute of Noetic Sciences, 1997)

6. Benson (1996) as cited in Newman, Robert Bruce *Calm Birth* (North Atlantic Books, 2006)

## CHAPTER SIX

1. Odent, Michel, *The Farmer and the Obstetrician* (Free Association Books, 2002)

2. Sikorski, J. 'A randomised controlled trial comparing two schedules of antenatal visits', *British Medical Journal* 312 (1996): 546–53; Villar, J. et al., 'WHO antenatal care randomised trial for the evaluation of a new model of routine antenatal care', *Lancet* 357 (2001): 1551–64; plus two more large-scale studies

3. Carolan, M., Nelson S., 'First mothering over 35 Years: questioning the Association of Maternal Age and Pregnancy Risk', *Health Care for Women International* 28 (2007): 534–55

4. Gerhardt, Sue, *Why Love Matters* (Routledge, 2008): 67

5. Steer, P., et al., 'Relation between maternal haemoglobin concentration and birth weight in different ethnic groups', *British Medical Journal* 310 (1995): 489–91; see also Odent, Michel, *Birth and Breastfeeding* (Clairview Books, 2007): xiii

6. Valberg L.S., 'Effects of iron, tin and copper on zinc absorption in humans', *American Journal of Clinical Nutrition* 40 (1984): 536–41

7. Odent, Michel op. cit: xv refers to four separate studies published in the *American Society of Obstetrics and Gynecology* and the *Journal of the Royal Society of Medicine*
8. Ibid.
9. Rousselot, Susan op cit.: 92
10. According to *March of Dimes* research
11. Lawrence Beech, Beverley and Robinson, Jean, 'Unsound Ultrasound', *AIMS* (2005)
12. Ibid.
13. Numerous studies confirm that scans do not improve perinatal outcome, even in high-risk pregnancies: Ewigman, B.G., *et al.*, 'Effect of prenatal ultrasound screening on perinatal outcome', *New England Journal of Medicine* 329 (1993): 821–27 (trial involving 15,000 women). Also see Odent, Michel (2007) op. cit.: xi, xii and xiii
14. Ibid.
15. Murkoff and Mazel op. cit.: 62

## CHAPTER SEVEN

1. Murphy Paul, Annie, *Origins* (Hay House, 2010); Hüther, Gerald and Krens, Inge, *Das Geheimnis der ersten neuen Monate* (Patmos, 2008)
2. Auhagen-Stephanos op. cit.
3. Odent, M., 'Eat sardines, be happy ... and sing', *Midwifery Today* 59 (2001): 19
4. Halldorsson, T. I., *et al.*, 'Intake of artificially sweetened soft drinks and risk of preterm delivery', *American Journal of Clinical Nutrition* 92 (2010): 626–33

# CHAPTER EIGHT

1. Conducted by Dr Lewis-Mehl Madronna, Psychiatric Department of the University of Vermont Medical School and Arizona School of Medicine, cited in Mongan, Marie, *Hypnobirthing* (Souvenir Press, 2009)
2. Dinsmore-Tuli, Uma, *Yoga for Pregnancy and Birth* (Teach Yourself, 2010)
3. Ibid.
4. Field, T., *et al.*, 'Pregnant women benefit from massage therapy', *Journal of Psychosomatic Obstetrics and Gynaecology* 20 (1999): 31–38
5. Field, T., 'Labour pain is reduced by massage therapy', *Journal of Psychosomatic Obstetrics and Gynaecology* 18: 286–91
6. Lawn, J.E., *et al.*, 'Kangaroo mother care to prevent neonatal deaths due to preterm birth complications', *International Journal of Epidemiology* 39 (2010): 144–54. The review examined 15 studies including three randomised controlled trials

# CHAPTER NINE

1. Information using various sources including Mongan, Marie op. cit.; Ina May Gaskin's website and articles in *Midwifery Today*
2. Block, Jennifer, *Pushed: The Truth About Childbirth and Modern Maternity Care* (Da Capo, 2007); Kitzinger, Sheila and Tew, Marjorie, *Safer Childbirth? A Critical History of Maternity Care* (Free Association Books, 1998)
3. Odent, Michel, *Birth and Breastfeeding* op. cit.: 73
4. As observed by Jean-Pierre Hallet, who spent years living with and studying the Pygmies

5. Various studies confirm this, including: Buitendijk, S. E., 'Perinatal mortality and morbidity in a nationwide cohort of 529,688 low-risk planned home and hospital births', *International Journal of Obstetrics and Gynaecology* 116.9 (2009): 1177–84

6. Tew, M., 'Do obstetric intranatal interventions make birth safer?' *British Journal of Obstetrics and Gynaecology* 93.7 (1986): 659–74

7. MacKenzie, I. Z. and Cooke, I. (2001), 'What is a reasonable time from decision-to-delivery by caesarean section?' *British Journal of Obstetrics and Gynaecology* 109, 5 (2002), 498–504

8. Bell, J., *et al.*, 'Can obstetric complications explain the high levels of obstetric interventions and maternity service use among older women?' *British Journal of Obstetrics and Gynaecology* 108 (2001): 910–18

9. Grant, J., Editor's choice, *British Journal of Obstetrics and Gynaecology* 108 (2001): 9

10. Figes, Kate, *Life After Birth* (Virago, 2008): 91

11. Research database for primal health, www.birthworks.org and Odent, Michel essay 'The long-term consequences of how we are born'

12. Ibid.

13. Odent, Michel *Birth and Breastfeeding* op. cit.: 1, 11 and 13, Odent refers to 15 different studies and cites an article in *The Lancet* that compared eight studies from around the world involving tens of thousands of births

## CHAPTER TEN

1. Amalgamated from various articles, books and websites such as babycentre.co.uk, mumsnet.com and swissmom.ch

2. Gopnik, Alison, *The Philosophical Baby* (Bodley Head, 2009)

3. Gerhardt, Sue, *Why Love Matters* (Routledge, 2008)
4. Gerhardt, Sue op. cit.: 38
5. Hills-Bonczyk, S. G. *et al.*, 'Women's experiences with breastfeeding longer than 12 months', *Birth* 21 (1994): 206–12; and *The Right Time* baby survey showed 8 per cent of later mothers didn't breastfeed, 49 per cent breastfed more than 6 months, 24 per cent over 12 months
6. Bartick, M. and Reinhold A., 'The Burden of Suboptimal Breastfeeding in the United States: A Pediatric Cost Analysis', *Pediatrics* 125.5 (2010): 1048–56
7. Bermúdez de Castro, José María, director *Centro Nacional de Investigación sobre Evolución Humana* (CENIEH) in an interview with EFE, October 11th, 2009
8. None of this is made up! I am in touch with the woman via email, but she'd rather remain anonymous
9. Virtue, Doreen, *The Crystal Children* (Hay House, 2003): 137
10. Burell, S. and Exley, C. 'There is (still) too much aluminium in infant formulas', *BMC Pediatrics* 10.1 (2010): 63
11. More, S., 'Confectionary consumption in childhood and adult violence', *British Journal of Psychiatry* 195 (2009): 366–67
12. Jackson, Deborah, *Three in a Bed* (Bloomsbury, 2003); Sunderland, Margot, *The Science of Parenting* (DK Adult, 2006)
13. Gerhardt, Sue op. cit.: 65
14. Becker, Robert, *The Body Electric* (William Morrow, 1998)

## CHAPTER ELEVEN

1. Survey of 2,000 mothers commissioned by *Mother and Baby* magazine (2004)
2. Herrick, H., 'Postpartum depression: who gets help? Results from the Colorado, New York, and North Carolina PRAMS Surveys 1997–1999', North Carolina State Center for Health Statistics Statistical Brief 24.

# Bibliography

## BOOKS

Aughagen-Stephanos, Ute, *Damit mein Baby bleibt* (Kösel Verlag, 2009)

Berger Gross, Jessica, *About What Was Lost* (Plume, Penguin Group, 2007)

Block, Jennifer, *Pushed* (Da Capo 2007)

Byam-Cook, Clare, *What to Expect When You're Breastfeeding* (Vermilion, 2006)

Cannon, Emma, *The Baby-Making Bible* (Rodale, 2010)

Chavarro, Jorge and Willett, Walter, *The Fertility Diet* (McGraw-Hill, 2007)

Cooper, James, *The Five Point Plan* (B. Jain Publishers, 2010)

Dinsmore-Tuli, Uma, *Yoga for Pregnancy and Birth* (Teach Yourself, 2010)

Dobbyn, Sarah, *The Fertility Diet* (Simon & Schuster, 2008)

Dooley, Michael, *Fit for Fertility* (Hodder & Stoughton, 2007)

Evennett, Karen, *Natural Mother and Baby* (Neal's Yard Press, 2008)

Figes, Kate, *Life After Birth* (Virago, 2008)

Freedman, Françoise Barbira, *Yoga for Pregnancy* (Dorling Kindersley, 2004)

Gerhardt, Sue, *Why Love Matters* (Routledge, 2008)

Glenville, Marilyn, *Getting Pregnant Faster* (Kyle Cathie, 2008) www.marilynglenville.com

Godridge, Tracey and Gallie, Martine, *How to be a Great Working Mum* (Foulsham, 2008)

Gopnik, Alison, *The Philosophical Baby* (Bodley Head, 2009)

Gordon, Yehudi, *Birth and Beyond* (Vermilion, 2002)

Hardyment, Christina, *Dream Babies* (Jonathan Cape, 1983)

Holzgreye, Brigitte, *300 Fragen zur Schwangerschaft* (Gräfe und Unzer, 2003)

Hüther, Gerald and Krens, Inge, *Das Geheimnis der ersten neun Monate* (Patmos, 2008)

Jackson, Deborah, *Three in a Bed* (Bloomsbury, 2003)

Liedloff, Jean, *The Continuum Concept* (Penguin, 1986)

Marti, James and Heather Burton, *Holistic Pregnancy and Childbirth* (John Wiley, 1999)

Mongan, Marie, *HypnoBirthing* (Souvenir Press, 2009)

Murkoff, Heidi and Sharon Mazel, *What to Expect When You're Expecting* (Simon & Schuster, 2008)

Murphy Paul, Annie, *Origins* (Hay House, 2010)

Odent, Michel, *Birth and Breastfeeding* (Clairview Books, 2007)

Rousselot, Susan, *Avoiding Miscarriage* (Sea Change Press, 2007)

Scher, Jonathan and Dix, Carol, *Preventing Miscarriage* (Harper Collins, 2005)

Shazzie, *Evie's Kitchen* (Rawcreation, 2008)

Smith, Jon, *The Bloke's Guide to Pregnancy* (Hay House, 2008)

Sunderland, Margot, *The Science of Parenting* (DK Adult 2006)

Virtue, Doreen, *The Crystal Children* (Hay House 2003)

Weschler, Toni, *Taking Charge of Your Fertility* (Vermilion, 2003)

West, Zita, *Zita West's Guide to Getting Pregnant* (Harper Thorsons, 2005)

Wood, Kate, *Raw Living* (Grub Street, 2007)

## DOCUMENTARY FILMS

*The Business of Being Born*
*Orgasmic Birth*
*Birth As We Know It*

# Index

# JOIN THE HAY HOUSE FAMILY

As the leading self-help, mind, body and spirit publisher in the UK, we'd like to welcome you to our family so that you can enjoy all the benefits our website has to offer.

 **EXTRACTS** from a selection of your favourite author titles

 **COMPETITIONS, PRIZES & SPECIAL OFFERS** Win extracts, money off, downloads and so much more

 **LISTEN** to a range of radio interviews and our latest audio publications

 **CELEBRATE YOUR BIRTHDAY** An inspiring gift will be sent your way

 **LATEST NEWS** Keep up with the latest news from and about our authors

 **ATTEND OUR AUTHOR EVENTS** Be the first to hear about our author events

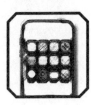 **iPHONE APPS** Download your favourite app for your iPhone

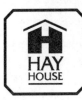 **HAY HOUSE INFORMATION** Ask us anything, all enquiries answered

## join us online at **www.hayhouse.co.uk**

 292B Kensal Road, London W10 5BE
T: 020 8962 1230 E: info@hayhouse.co.uk

# ABOUT THE AUTHOR

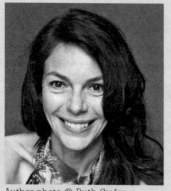

Author photo © Ruth Crafer

**Claudia Spahr** was born in York-shire to Swiss parents. She en-joyed a northern town childhood before leaving the rolling hills of Bronte-land, at age 15, for the al-pine pastures of Switzerland. She began her studies at Berne Univer-sity and then returned to the UK, where she completed a BA in Writ-ing and Publishing with Film and Literary Studies.

Claudia began a media career at the BBC German Service in London and then trained as a journalist with Swiss Radio International back in Berne. Having acquired a solid foundation in news and current af-fairs she switched to Swiss National Television where she spent a few years racing around the country as a reporter. In Zurich they decided she had enough cheek to become a foreign correspondent and sent her to cover the UK and Ireland – where she became in effect 'The London office'.

After ten years in radio and TV, Claudia decided to change her life-style. She based herself in Cambodia to work on a novel, *She Nomads*, and completed the manuscript in Vietnam and New York. Together with her Spanish partner, Claudia also set up a yoga and healing resort on the beach in South Goa, India. She is now juggling mother-hood with being a full-time author.